T0271619

THE 20 Minute Gut Health Fix

super simple recipes to supercharge your health + avoid ultra-processed food

Dr Saliha Mahmood Ahmed

PHOTOGRAPHY BY STEVE JOYCE

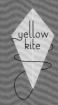

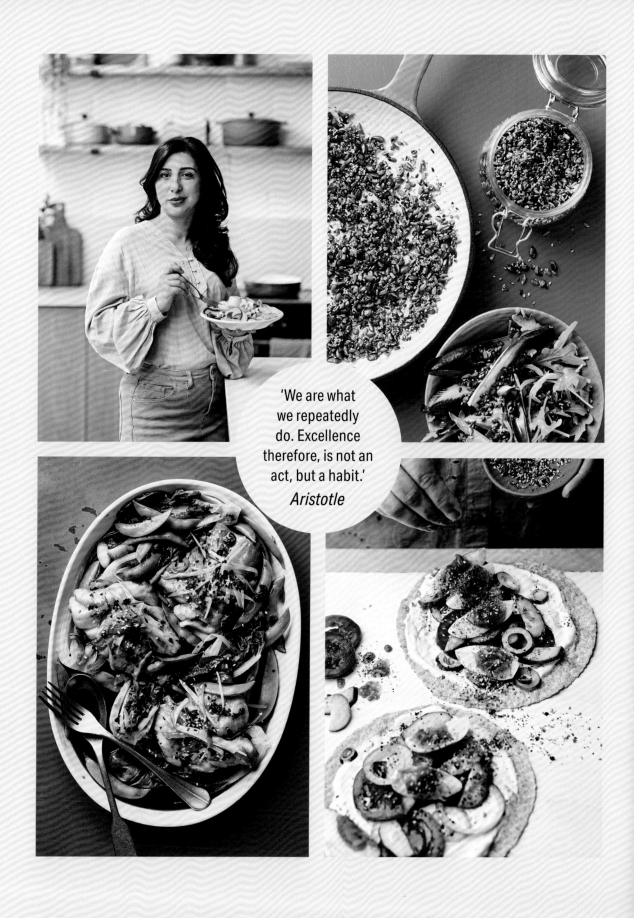

'We are what we repeatedly do. Excellence therefore, is not an act, but a habit.'
Aristotle

Contents

Introduction

Imagine someone from a hundred years ago travels forward in time and asks you to explain modern life to them. You would tell them that by picking up a small rectangular device you could, in a matter of seconds, speak to anyone in any other part of the world. That by typing a few words into said device, milliseconds later you would have an avalanche of knowledge at your disposal. The time traveller would be completely awestruck at the speed with which we now function.

When we take a step back it is clear that the lightning pace of modern life is nothing short of miraculous. But in a world where everything, including time itself, feels accelerated, the constant flow of information can leave us feeling overloaded and stressed. The perpetual dizziness that this time pressure creates leaves little time or tolerance for slower pursuits – like cooking.

With the demands of work, family, friends, cleaning the house, doing the shopping, not to mention finding any sliver of time for self-care, our lives often pull us in ten different directions at once. And if we do miraculously manage to get on top of all those other pressures, it's not often that we will use our precious remaining energy hunched over a stove.

As a gastroenterologist and chef, this breaks my heart. Patients tell me the same thing time and time again: 'I just don't have time to cook!' This is nobody's fault; it's just how life is these days. In the past, I have been just as guilty of demoting cooking to the 'maybe tomorrow' pile. This book is my way of trying to change the status quo, to turn the creation of great food from a time-consuming chore to a fun, express 20-minute activity.

What we choose to eat has such a direct impact on our long-term health (both mental and physical) that it pains me to think that 21st-century life is slowly eroding cooking from our lives in favour of ready meals and takeaways.

SO, HOW DO WE REBRAND COOKING?

I want everyone who reads this book to leave with the knowledge that in this world full of multinational food conglomerates pushing ultra-processed food into our diets, and social media overload making it impossible to separate fact from misinformation, gut-healthy home-cooked food can be slick and sexy.

One big problem we face is that technological advancement has far outpaced social customs and the norms around cooking. Find any cookbook in your kitchen and open it to a random page. How long does the recipe take to cook from start to finish? An hour? Two? More? While some chefs are beginning to recognise that long cook times are just not feasible in today's busy households, too many published recipes still have multiple steps, excess ingredients and multi-hour preparation and cooking times. These cookbooks are often more about aspiration than practicality.

The key is convenience. For any given mealtime, whether that is breakfast, brunch, lunch, dinner or the snacks in between, this book is here to prove to you that you can get gut-healthy, vibrant, appetising food on your table within minutes of walking into the kitchen. This is the ultimate low effort, high reward outcome: dishes that contribute positively and substantially to the health of you and your family, but that don't

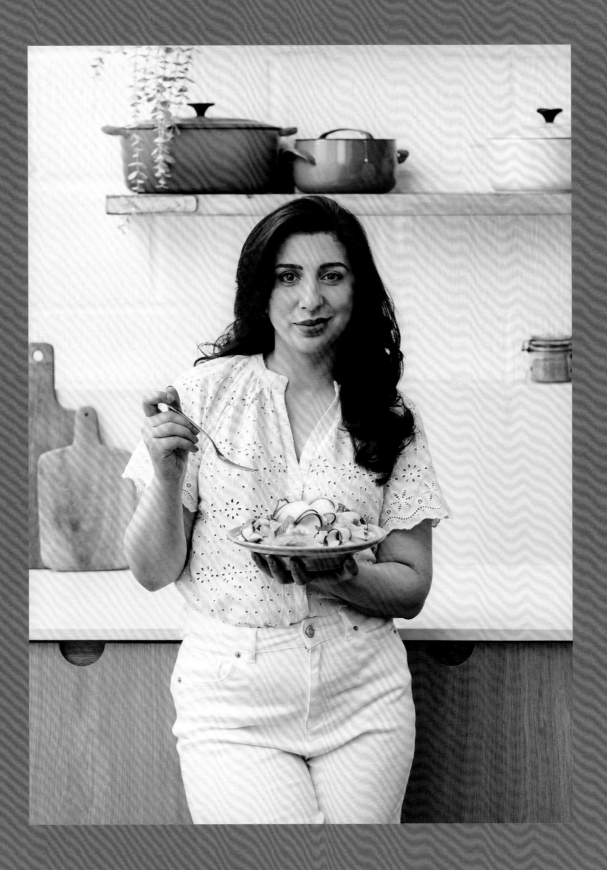

Prioritising the health of your gut bacteria is one of the most important choices a person can make.

take huge amounts of time or money to create. Of course, I do recognise the appeal of a slow-cooked pot of deliciousness, and there certainly is a time and place for it. But it's the recipes that taste great relative to the effort required to make them that have become the beloved staples that I turn to time and again. And when I think of my two boys, it's definitely the quick recipes that they want to help me cook, and that they ask for again and again and again.

The uniqueness of this book lies in the fact that all the recipes should take no more than 20 minutes to make. I have practised them over and over again, with my husband and children serving as willing judges and eager sous chefs; I can confidently say that they have consistently clocked in under the magic 20-minute mark.

In keeping with my other books, these recipes are based on the principles of gut-healthy eating. This isn't just a buzzword or a fad; from my knowledge and experience as a gastroenterologist I can tell you that prioritising the health of your gut bacteria is one of the most important choices a person can make. What's more, gut-friendly food choices can result in tangible improvements in key aspects of your health long into the future. Weight loss, diabetes prevention, reduction of cardiovascular disease risk and better mental health can all be achieved by reconsidering what's on your plate.

When I wrote my last cookbook, *The Kitchen Prescription*, I wasn't sure what sort of reception it would get. Most cookbooks don't spend time discussing how probiotics can positively impact the frequency and consistency of our poo before launching into a recipe! But my goodness, I have been completely bowled over by the number of

positive messages from readers, telling me about real tangible differences to their health outcomes that they have noticed since using my recipes.

With this new collection of recipes I want to continue this journey with you, so that you are levelling up your cooking repertoire in a way that deliberately and intentionally benefits those billions of tireless gut inhabitants that keep you going, day in, day out. However, before we get to any recipes, I want to guide you through some of the core principles of what gut-healthy eating entails, as well as take you through what's at the opposite end of the scale: ultra-processed foods. We'll look at why we seem to be so reliant on them, and what we can do to reverse this reliance with minimal effort and inconvenience.

Finally, I'll be walking you through a guided reflection on your own personal circumstances and eating behaviours, so that any dietary changes that you decide to make after reading these recipes can be focused and sustainable for the long term.

Humans are unique in that we are the only species that has discovered the joy of cooking. Heating our ingredients to change their molecular structure has opened up a whole world of nutrition, taste and texture that literally no other species on earth can access by themselves. Life is about food, living for it and through it. The sights and sounds of the chop, sizzle and roast, the joy of the first bite of something utterly delicious. Sometimes we forget about the pleasure that comes from creating food, but I believe it's one of the purest forms of mortal happiness there is. So, let's use this skill that only we possess, and get gut-healthy. Only this time, we have just 20 minutes!

Introduction

What is Gut Healthy Eating?

Gut-healthy eating is – thankfully – no fleeting trend and so many more of us are now appreciating the importance of gut health to our overall wellbeing. However, while there is currently a lot of hype around gut health, a basic knowledge of what it actually means can be patchy or inadequate for many. This chapter will, I hope, bring you up to speed with the fundamentals.

The gut is a complex system of unimaginable intricacy, able to communicate with virtually every part of the body through the actions of nerves, hormones and the immune system. Our gut is home to the microbiota, a gargantuan mass of around a hundred trillion or more microbes, aka 'bugs'. These gut bugs began their development when we passed through our mother's vaginal canal and, in most adults, have a combined weight of over 2kg/4lb.

Our gut bugs possess their own set of genes that are collectively called the microbiome. The genes which make up the gut microbiome are vast, outnumbering our mere 23,000 or so human genes; some estimates put the number of genes in the gut microbiome at 22,000,000. And thanks to the marvels of modern technology, a simple stool test is all it takes to map the gut microbiome.

Each person's gut microbiome is like their own unique fingerprint: your microbiome will never be like anyone else in the world. In simple terms, we need to cultivate and nurture our gut bugs because the more diverse our population of gut bugs, the better it is for our overall health. Studies have shown that our risk of developing heart disease and stroke, diabetes, Parkinson's disease, inflammatory bowel disease, obesity and even certain cancers is influenced by the composition of our gut microbiota.

A healthy, diverse gut microbiota is an ecological entity, capable of producing thousands of metabolites, which can influence the levels of inflammation and 'leakiness' of the gut wall and can even alter the sensitivity of the gut to insulin, the hormone that controls blood sugar and lipids. Our gut microbes can produce enzymes and vitamins that we can't make ourselves or get directly from our diet. They can even help us break down otherwise indigestible nutrients from our food.

When you stop to think about this it's completely astounding: billions of individual organisms working as one inside your body to help you digest and make the most of that Weetabix you had for breakfast. Eighteen years ago, when I started medical school, not a single word was uttered about the impact of gut bugs on health. None of us even knew the word microbiome. But things are changing – slowly.

Contrary to what some companies claim, what we cannot do at this moment in time is look at the composition of an individual's gut microbiome and give specific advice on what they should be eating to optimise their health. Currently, this is beyond the capabilities of reliable science, so be wary of unscrupulous wellness companies and their big promises. As a gastroenterologist, I have had patients come to me with printouts of their microbiome composition, asking me what it means and what to do; this is advice that I am simply not able to give. Right now, there are still too many unknowns. However, we aren't that far off; the realm of 'precision medicine', where personalised, tailored nutrition advice can be offered to patients is, thanks to cutting-edge science, nearer than we think.

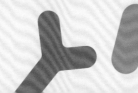

How to Develop a Healthy Internal Eco System

What we *can* do is use the most up-to-date evidence to guide people on the principles of what foods and eating patterns will help foster a healthy internal ecosystem. I can also share the most delicious recipes to inspire you and keep your gut microbiome ticking over smoothly.

EAT MORE PLANTS

It really is that simple. There is no magic bullet to developing a healthy microbiome. No potion or supplement can achieve what a diet full of plants can. In gut-health circles, a diet where over 30 different plants are eaten on average in the course of a week is probably the most beneficial action we can take to optimise gut health.

Hang on. Did I say 30 different plants a week? I'm not even sure I could name 30 different plants. Worry not, readers. Achieving plant diversity is not actually as daunting as it may sound. By plants, I don't mean that you need to start nibbling on the shrubs and grasses growing in your back garden, in fact all of the below count as plants.

1. Fruits and Vegetables
2. Wholegrains
3. Legumes and Pulses
4. Nuts and Seeds
5 Spices and Herbs

Before you dismiss this book as just another plant-based cookbook, I would like to clarify that I am neither a vegetarian nor a vegan, nor is this cookbook. What I am is a great advocate of what I refer to as 'plant-centricity' or 'plant-forward eating', because eating more plants really is the key for us to have any chance of improving our gut health. And remember, it's not just about eating more plants, it's about eating a wider, more diverse range of plants. If your diet contains plants of every colour of the rainbow, you're doing something right. To help you increase the variety of plants in your diet, each recipe in this book contains a 'diversity score'. This score is simply the number of plant portions the recipe contains, and you can use this to track your progress towards the 30 plants per week target.

The more sceptical among you may be asking, why 30? Why not 25 or 50 plants per week, or some other random number? Great question! It's based on research that emerged in 2018 as part of the American Gut Project, where an analysis of 10,000 samples of stool showed that the people who ate 30 or more plants a week were far more likely to have certain 'good bugs' than those who ate just 10 plants a week.

In practice, I have found that 30 a week, although it sounds daunting, is actually a feasible target for most people to work towards. Notice I said 'work towards' and not 'achieve immediately'. To begin with, you are likely to be making health gains by increasing the number of plant points from your baseline; for example, if you currently eat five different plant foods per week, you might finish the first few weeks on 10 different plant foods, which is a great achievement! The target is an end goal, designed to encourage you to eat more of the good stuff. It's not meant to be a source of anxiety, stress or feelings of failure.

A big reason why a rainbow of plants is good for our gut health is because plants offer our gut bacteria a variety of dietary fibre and polyphenolic compounds, which they love. Polyphenols are processed and converted by our gut bugs to

PORTION SIZE

There are no exact serving sizes for plant portions, but as a rule of thumb I would say the following . . .

1 portion
=

A handful for fruit and veg, wholegrains, legumes and pulses

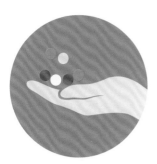

1 portion
=

Half a handful for nuts, seeds and herbs

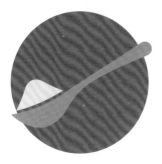

1 portion
=

A teaspoon for spices.

beneficial 'bioactive' compounds, leading to the enhanced proliferation of the 'good' bugs and a relative decrease in the number of 'bad' bugs that promote inflammation.

The concept of plant-centric eating is not new. What's new is our deepened understanding of how beneficial plants are to gut health, which has resulted in us packaging the 'more plants = better' message in a new way. For example, if you cast your eye over the famous Eatwell Guide, it clearly has a strong emphasis on including more plants in our diets. The '5 a day' campaign is also a direct attempt at promoting plant-centricity in our diets. And the maths savvy among you might have noticed that there's not that much difference between 30 a week and 5 a day (provided it's not the same 5 a day every day); after all, the approaches all share a common goal, which is to promote an achievable target for us to aim for when increasing our plant intake.

A benefit of eating more plants is that (relative to fresh meat and poultry) plants are substantially cheaper. Tinned and frozen vegetables, legumes, pulses and dried grains are fantastically inexpensive and have an incredibly long shelf life.

But let's not beat around the bush: buying fresh produce and a range of different plants is expensive, and for many people unattainable. In 2023, the Broken Plate report showed that for those families on low-income backgrounds, a massive 50 per cent of their disposable income would have to be spent on food to mirror the Eatwell Guide's recommendations.

And it's reasons like this that begin to tell us why ultra-processed foods are so prolific; 200g (7oz) of mixed nuts cost around £3.50, which is about the same as 12 packets of crisps. I know what I would be forced to choose if I was on a limited budget. with kids to feed, and it's not the nuts. At a time when the cost of everything is skyrocketing, from mortgages and rent to utility bills, it is clear that affordability of food and ingredients will be an important consideration for many using this book. I have tried to be mindful of this when designing these recipes.

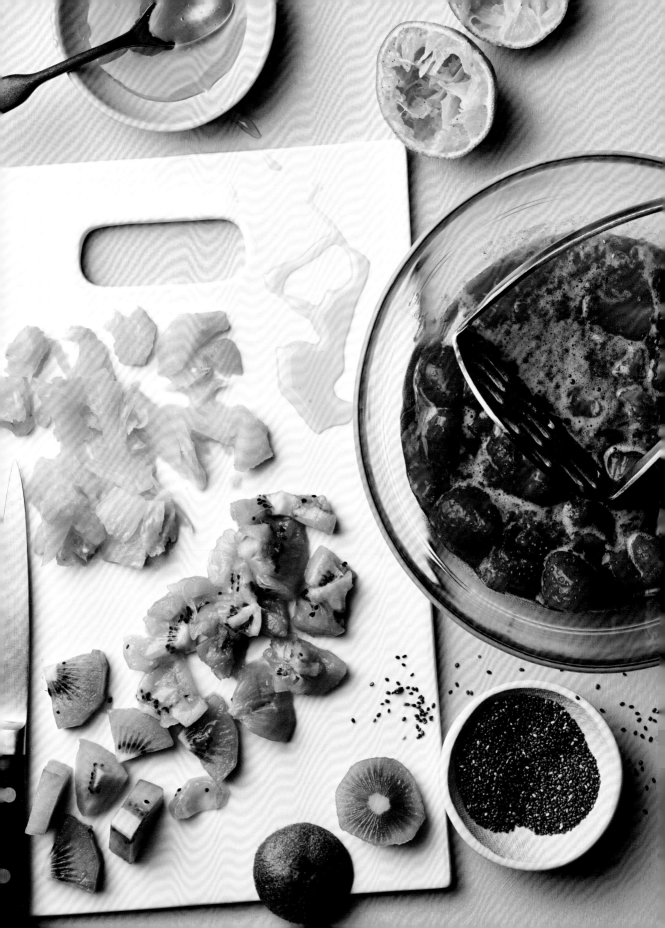

The Dos of Gut-Healthy Eating

To foster a healthy relationship with food, no one food or food group should be demonised. There is a role for all food in our diets, from the healthiest salad to the gooiest chocolate cake, and labelling entire groups of food as 'good' or 'bad', attaching some kind of moral value to them and trying to shame people into removing certain foods from their diets is at best unhelpful and at worst dangerous.

DO EAT PREBIOTICS + PROBIOTIC FOODS

Prebiotic and probiotic foods have become synonymous with gut health but while awareness and interest in these foods is expanding, the reality is that most of us don't actually know the difference between the two. Here's what you need to know:

• Prebiotic foods

These are the fertilisers that we apply to our gut. These foods are rich in fibre, which encourages the beneficial growth and proliferation of our gut microbes. The fibre in prebiotic foods has to be strong enough to not be broken down by our stomach acids or the digestive enzymes thrown at them in the small intestine. They reach the colon whole where our gut bugs ferment them, producing beneficial compounds that our body needs to stay in tip top health. Some popular proven prebiotics include whole grains, apples, bananas, leeks, asparagus, cauliflower, broccoli, chicory, honey, garlic, seeds nuts, lentils, peas, tomato and rye.

• Probiotic foods

These are the seeds that we plant in our gut in the hope that new species will flourish. Probiotic foods actually contain live bugs and aim to restore bacterial balance; the theory is that a probiotic food will resist the action of acid and enzymes to eventually reach the colon, where it will make its home, have many more bacterial babies, and change the overall gut microbial composition for the better.

Technically speaking, to classify as a probiotic a food item must confer some proven benefit to health, but many foods labelled as probiotics are in actual fact just fermented foods where the health benefit, while likely, remains unproven.

I use probiotic foods like live yoghurt, kefir, kimchi (a personal favourite) and sauerkraut liberally in my cooking, but it's also fun to use lesser-known probiotics like lacto-fermented turnips, carrots, cucumbers or jalapeños and olives fermented in brine and miso paste. These foods taste slightly 'funky', adding a lactic twang and a huge amount of depth to your dishes. I encourage you to experiment with these incredible ingredients because they will almost certainly do a healthy person no harm and may well do you some good.

Most of the evidence suggests that prebiotic and probiotic ingredients work together to create their immense health benefits, and so it's impossible to decide which one is more important overall. A probiotic is unlikely to be as beneficial in an environment where there are no prebiotic fibres to help them flourish. But if you don't like the taste of probiotics, don't sweat. Just get as many prebiotics into the diet as possible and fertilise that gut!

EVALUATE YOUR FIBRE INTAKE

While I have never been one to encourage people to obsessively count nutrients, I do think our fibre intake might be the one thing to keep an eye on. Technically, fibre is not considered a nutrient because it isn't absorbed by the body but fibre really is the forgotten nutritional hero. It's one of the most powerful health-promoting ingredients we know of, yet one that our classic Western diets have shamefully neglected. When our gut microbes get to work fermenting fibre, the short-chain fatty acids that are produced have proven beneficial effects on our health, such as a reduction of the risk of heart disease and stroke, type 2 diabetes and bowel cancer. There are also short-term benefits to increasing fibre intake; I meet countless patients with chronic constipation and the vast majority see huge improvements in their bowel function when they introduce more fibre in their diets. The target for adults is 30g of fibre per day, but in the UK many people are only getting around one third of that. Think back to what you ate yesterday; if you start counting you may be surprised by how little fibre you actually eat on a daily basis. The recipes in this book have been designed to help you incorporate more fibre into your diet, something that I know from experience can be a significant challenge. To help you out, the fibre content per portion is listed for each recipe, giving you an easy way to keep an eye on how much fibre you are eating per day. Can you hit that magic 30g?

Fibre is divided into soluble and insoluble varieties, and ideally what we are looking for in our diets is a mix of the two. The ideal ratio will differ from person to person, since it appears that different fibre combinations suit different people. As their names suggest, soluble fibres dissolve in water and break down into a gel-like substance, while insoluble fibres don't dissolve in water. The table opposite is a guide so you can get an idea of the amount of soluble and insoluble fibre various common foods contain.

DO DRINK COFFEE (MAYBE WITH A SQUARE OF DARK CHOCOLATE)

This is good news if, like me, you love a nice cup of coffee in the morning. It might be the effect of vitamins and minerals in the coffee beans, or perhaps the fact that coffee is a mixture of soluble fibres that have some prebiotic properties. Whatever it is, coffee is helpful for our gut microbiota.

Consider this next time you sip your brew:
- *Research suggests that the antioxidant properties of coffee may help repair damaged cells and therefore reduce the risk of developing some cancers, Parkinson's and even Alzheimer's disease.*
- *Coffee contains chlorogenic acid, which may have valuable metabolic benefits, helping reduce the risk of diabetes and obesity.*
- *Coffee directly stimulates the gastrocolic reflex; around a third of us will feel a powerful urge to poo after a strong cup of coffee, which is great for anyone suffering from chronic constipation.*

Let's not forget, though, that despite all these benefits coffee is also a source of caffeine and so it is important to be aware of your body and your personal limits. While coffee is likely to be very beneficial to gut health, those benefits might be reversed if you are up all night and your sleep is impacted.

But what about that square of chocolate? Dark chocolate that has few other ingredients and upwards of 70 per cent cocoa solids can give you 8–9g of fibre per 100g (by contrast, milk chocolate has just 2–3g per 100g). Good-quality dark chocolate is also rich in vitamins, minerals, antioxidants and polyphenols. So basically, what I'm saying is that coffee and dark chocolate together are a match made in gut health heaven.

FOOD SOURCES OF FIBRE

Food	Serving Size	Total Fibre (*grams*)	Soluble Fibre (*grams*)	Insoluble Fibre (*grams*)
FRUIT				
Apple, with skin	1 medium	3.3	0.4	2.9
Banana	1 medium	3.1	2.2	0.9
Pear, with skin	1 medium	5.2	1.1	4.1
Orange	1 medium	3.2	2.1	1.1
Prunes	¼ cup	4.6	2.5	2.1
Raspberries	½ cup	4.0	1.2	2.8
Strawberries	½ cup	1.7	0.4	1.3
VEGETABLES				
Asparagus	½ cup	1.8	0.3	1.5
Broccoli, cooked	½ cup	2.6	0.3	2.3
Brussels sprouts, cooked	½ cup	3.2	1.1	2.1
Carrots	1 large	2.0	0.9	1.1
Potato, baked with skin	1 medium	4.4	1.1	3.3
Spinach, cooked	½ cup	2.2	0.7	1.5
BEANS, LEGUMES, NUTS + SEEDS				
Black beans, cooked	½ cup	7.5	2.1	5.4
Butter beans, cooked	½ cup	5.4	1.5	3.9
Chickpeas, cooked	½ cup	5.3	1.3	4.0
Green peas, cooked	⅔ cup	5.7	2.3	3.4
Kidney beans, cooked	½ cup	5.7	2.3	3.4
Lentils, cooked	⅔ cup	10.4	1.7	8.7
Pinto beans, cooked	½ cup	7.7	3.3	3.4
Peanut butter, chunky	2 tbsp	2.6	0.7	1.9
Psyllium seeds, ground	1 tbsp	6.0	5.0	1.0
WHOLE GRAINS				
Barley, cooked	½ cup	6.8	1.4	5.4
Brown rice, cooked ½ cup	½ cup	1.8	0.2	1.6
English muffin (wholewheat)	1	4.4	1.3	3.1
Rolled oats, cooked ¾ cup	¾ cup	4.2	2.0	2.2
Wholewheat bread 1 slice	1 slice	2.8	0.4	2.4

A note of caution: If you increase your fibre intake, make sure you do it slowly. Take it from a gastroenterologist who has seen it all; increasing fibre too quickly can lead to excessive bloating, flatulence and abdominal discomfort. Slow and steady wins the fibre race.

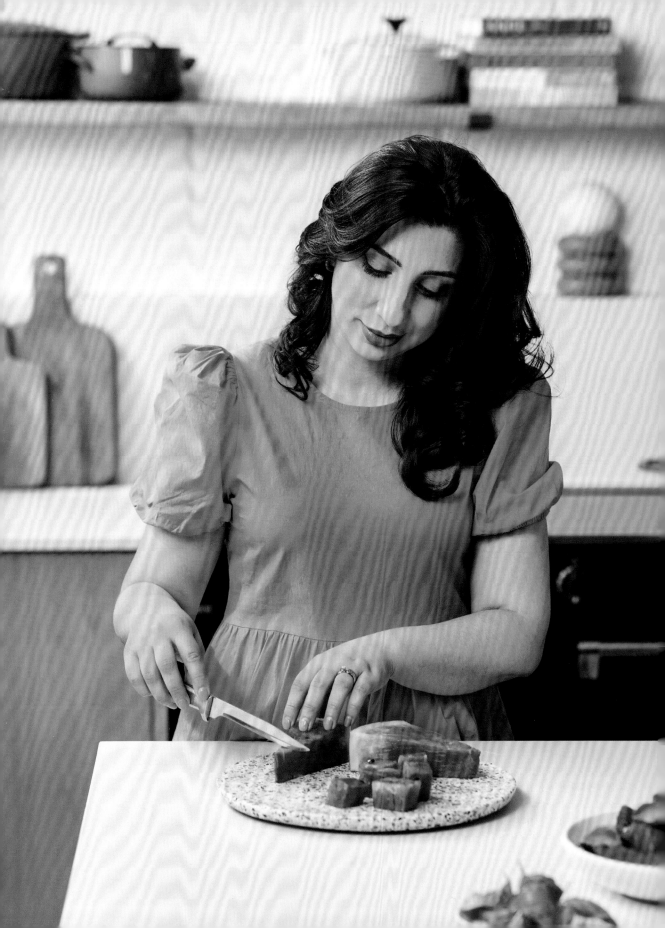

DO TRY TO GET SOME OMEGA-3 FATS INTO YOUR DIET

Doctors and researchers spend a lot of time and energy looking at the impact of fibre on the composition of our gut bugs. But in contrast, we spend very little time looking at the impact that other things like fat have on our gut. This seems like a significant oversight as we know that some fats like omega-3 are anti-inflammatory. These fats have also been linked consistently to better heart health, reduced chronic inflammation, reduced heart disease, reduced type 2 diabetes and even lowered risk of depression.

Even more promising, a few studies looking into the effects of omega-3 fats on health have suggested that they may also be directly helpful for the health of our microbiome, although the research here is still in its early stages. Salmon, herring, mackerel, tuna and sardines are all cold-water fatty fish rich in beneficial omega-3 fats (docosahexaenoic acid and eicosapentaenoic acid, for anyone interested). Plant sources of omega-3 (alpha linolenic acid) include flaxseeds or their oil, chia seeds, walnuts and rapeseed oil. Long-term studies of certain populations suggest that people who have diets rich in omega-3 fats (such as the Italians) enjoy a lowered risk from heart disease.

I use both cold-water oily fish and plant sources of omega-3 throughout this book. If you're looking for a healthy dose of this important anti-inflammatory fat, try the Kimchi and Mackerel Kedgeree (page 79), Tuna, Quinoa and Ginger Fishcakes (page 177) or Five-Minute Overnight Oats (page 48).

DO HAVE AS MUCH PLANT PROTEIN AS POSSIBLE

Plants contain valuable proteins, and while they are not 'complete' sources of all the amino acids by themselves, a good variety of plants in your diet will allow you to meet your protein requirements and get all the amino acids you need with relative ease. Now, please don't feel that I'm telling you to become a vegetarian or a vegan. I still enjoy meat, poultry and fish in moderation and feel the pain of those who want to cut back on the amount of meat they eat but find it a struggle. I myself come from a culture where meat is celebrated and forms the basis of most meals, but the more I learn about this topic, the more I am convinced that significantly lowering our meat consumption and simultaneously boosting the amount of plants we eat is the way forward.

Here are some small changes that might help transition from less animal to more plant protein:

- *If you use processed meat (ham, bacon, corned beef, sausages, etc.) in your recipes, cut down your portion size or see if you can find an unprocessed alternative.*

- *However corny they might sound, try a 'Meat Free Monday' or 'Vegnesday' or make a 'Veg Pledge' with colleagues or family members.*

- *Try substituting legumes, pulses, beans or lentils in place of meat in your usual dishes.*

Processed meat in particular contains nitrates and nitrites, which can cause damage to the cell lining of the gut wall. Eating lots of processed meat and red meat has also been linked to increased risk of developing bowel cancer.

How the gut microbiota is impacted by meat intake has not yet been thoroughly studied, but the general consensus is that processed meat might contribute to a microbial environment that corresponds to high levels of intestinal inflammation. By cutting down overall meat consumption and replacing it with plant protein sources not only can you improve your gut health, you can also reduce your personal carbon footprint and enjoy meat in a more sustainable way, which is a win in anyone's book.

What is Ultra Processed Food?

The easiest way to think about ultra-processed food is to think about sweetcorn. There's nothing quite like a sweet, juicy corn on the cob straight out of the pot. But what about a packet of cheese puffs? These addictive snacks look nothing like corn, taste nothing like corn, but they did, in fact, start out as corn kernels. They are the result of extensive processing to turn a natural corn kernel into an air-filled crunchy puff.

Thousands of foods that we consume are processed in many hundreds of different ways: to add flavour, taste and texture, to make them more digestible, to make them safe to consume, to give them a longer shelf life, or just to make them look more attractive on the supermarket shelf. Even if you cook most of your meals from scratch, chances are you'll be using many ingredients that have been processed in some way, like tinned tomatoes and pulses or olive oil. A 'processed' food is one that is not used in its raw state. Anything we do to food, from baking to boiling, roasting to microwaving and air frying, is all applying 'process' to food.

However, nobody would argue that tinned lentils are unhealthy just because they've been 'processed'. So what's the difference between a processed food and an ultra-processed food (UPF)? As the name suggests, ultra-processed foods lie at the extreme end of the processed food spectrum and have been the subject of a huge amount of debate and media interest over the last few years.

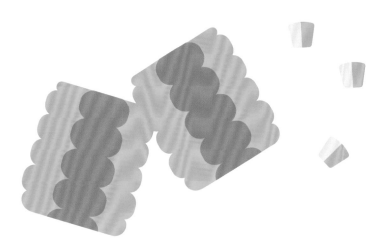

HOW TO IDENTIFY AN ULTRA-PROCESSED FOOD

If you were to guess, how much of your diet do you think consists of ultra-processed foods? Ten per cent? Twenty? Shockingly, research suggests that in the UK today around 57 per cent of an adult's diet and around 80 per cent of a child's diet is made up of UPFs. Worryingly, these are among the highest figures in Europe.

Despite us eating such huge amounts of UPFs, recent surveys suggest that only 4 in 10 of us understand the term 'ultra-processed' correctly, while only 1 in 10 think about the level of processing in the food items we buy.

A good way to gauge how processed a food item is, is to look at the ingredients list. Generally speaking, the longer the ingredient list is for any given food item, the more likely it is to sit firmly at the ultra-processed end of the food spectrum. Another clue is to look for items that you wouldn't find in your own kitchen store cupboard. The following are items that are regularly added to UPFs:

1. Protein sources
   (hydrolysed proteins, soya protein isolate, gluten, casein, whey protein, mechanically separated meat).

2. Sugars
   (fructose, high-fructose corn syrup, fruit juice concentrates, invert sugar, maltodextrin, dextrose, lactose.)

3. Modified oils
   (hydrogenated oil and interesterified oil).

4. Additives
   (flavours, flavour enhancers, colours, emulsifiers, emulsifying salts, sweeteners, thickeners, and anti-foaming, bulking, carbonating, foaming, gelling and glazing agents).

A long ingredients list doesn't always mean that the food is definitely going to be a UPF, but it's an incredibly good indication. But is there something a bit more scientific, like a classification system, to tell us what is and what isn't a UPF? Luckily, there is! The NOVA classification system was developed in Brazil by Professor Carlos Monteiro. It categorises processing into four groups, with Group 1 being the least processed and Group 4 being the most processed.

THE NOVA CLASSIFICATION SYSTEM

Group 1

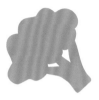

- <u>Unprocessed or minimally processed foods</u>

  > Fresh, dry or frozen vegetables or fruit, grains, legumes, meat, fish, eggs, nuts and seeds.

  > Processing includes removal of edible/unwanted parts. Does not add substances to the original food.

Group 2

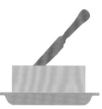

- <u>Processed culinary ingredients</u>

  > Plant oils (e.g. olive oil, coconut oil), animal fats (e.g. cream, butter, lard), maple syrup, sugar, honey and salt.

  > Substances derived from Group 1 foods or from nature by processes including pressing, refining, grinding, milling and drying.

Group 3

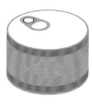

- <u>Processed Food</u>

  > Tinned/pickled vegetables, meat, fish or fruit, artisanal bread, cheese, salted meats, wine, beer and cider.

  > Processing of foods from Group 1 or 2 with the addition of oil, salt or sugar by means of tinning, pickling, smoking, curing or fermentation.

Group 4

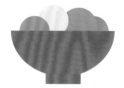

- <u>Ultra-processed foods</u>

  > Sugar-sweetened beverages, sweet and savoury packaged snacks, reconstituted meat products, pre-prepared frozen dishes, tinned/instant soups, chicken nuggets, ice cream.

  > Formulations made from a series of processes including extraction and chemical modification. Includes very little intact Group 1 foods.

Look at the example below of two SHOP BOUGHT CRACKERS, which look similar, but have very different ingredients. These illustrate the difference between ultra-processed and non-ultra-processed food items. Once you start looking, you will notice really stark differences in the ingredients lists across products.

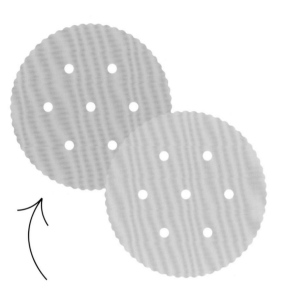

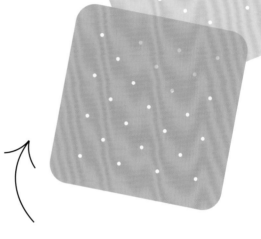

ULTRA-PROCESSED CRACKERS

These crackers contain emulsifer, soy lecithin and natural flavour. They also have high fructose corn syrup, a sweetner made from corn starch. This is a key ingredient in fizzy drinks and sweets.

NON ULTRA-PROCESSED CRACKERS

These crackers have 3 ingredients: wholegrain wheat, canola oil and sea salt.

INGREDIENTS
UNBLEACHED ENRICHED FLOUR (WHEAT FLOUR, NIACIN, REDUCED IRON, THIAMINE MONONITRATE {VITAMIN B1}, RIBOFLAVIN {VITAMIN B2}, FOLIC ACID), SOYBEAN AND/OR CANOLA OIL, PALM OI, SUGAR, SALT, LEAVENING (CALCIUM PHOSPHATE, BAKING SODA) HIGH FRUCTOSE CORN SYRUP, SOY LECITHIN, NATURAL FLAVOUR.

CONTAINS:
WHEAT, SOY

INGREDIENTS
WHOLE GRAIN WHEAT, CANOLA OIL, SEA SALT.

CONTAINS:
WHEAT

ARE ULTRA-PROCESSED FOODS 'BAD' FOR US?

According to a study of over 200,000 adults across four different countries, increasing calorie intake from ultra-processed foods by just 10 per cent is associated with a 15 per cent higher risk of 'all-cause mortality'. In simple terms, eating more ultra-processed foods can cause an early death.

Most recently, in 2024, an even bigger Australian study that looked at the eating patterns of a whopping 10 million people found that there is an undeniable association between ultra-processed foods and risk of cardiovascular disease, common mental health disorders, type 2 diabetes and mortality. But there is an important distinction to make here: the association between UPFs and these health outcomes does not mean causality. As yet we don't have clear evidence that it is the processing of food that directly causes the damage to our health.

But just because we cannot prove with 100 per cent certainty that UPFs are the cause of the negative health outcomes observed, does not mean that the correlation should be ignored. The scale of the problem is huge and potential harm is of colossal magnitude. Scientists have therefore recommended – and rightly so – that governments take urgent action to reduce the number of UPFs that we consume.

The NOVA classification is quite broad and encompasses a huge number of foods that are high in sugar, salt and fat and have poor nutritional content. We understand exactly how high levels of sugar, fat and salt can lead to negative health outcomes, but it's much harder to pin down exactly how processing leads to these problems. In the example of the cheesy corn puff, is it the fact that the maize plant has been processed to the extent that its food matrix is altered that makes it bad for us, or is it the high fat and salt that are driving the problem? In science, mechanisms really do matter.

There is a huge drive to find out exactly what it is about UPFs that makes them harmful. This is a space to watch carefully as exciting research is on the horizon.

What we have observed is that ultra-processed foods seem to have a negative effect on our gut microbes, and this is possibly because of the lack of fibre in almost all UPFs. Whether the UPF comes from an animal or plant source doesn't seem to make much difference; both types seem to impact our gut inhabitants negatively. So unfortunately, in terms of our gut health there isn't much difference between an ultra-processed sausage roll and an ultra-processed vegan sausage roll.

One thing I've noticed, and that I want to try to avoid in this book, is the complete demonisation of ultra-processed foods. People eat UPFs for a number of reasons, be it preference, budget, convenience, time constraints, or any number of other equally valid considerations. Attaching a moral value to foods based on their level of processing completely ignores the valid reasons for their existence, and by shaming people for choosing to eat them we can unconsciously cause significant damage to an individual's mental health and their overall relationship with food.

Similarly, tarring all ultra-processed foods with the same brush runs the risk of unintended harmful consequences. For example, wholegrain cereals are classed as ultra-processed, but if we removed them from the supermarket shelves, we would also be removing the many key vitamins and minerals that they are fortified with, as well as an incredibly useful and abundant source of dietary fibre.

Scientists have recommended that governments take urgent action to reduce the number of UPFs that we consume.

What is Ultra Processed Food?

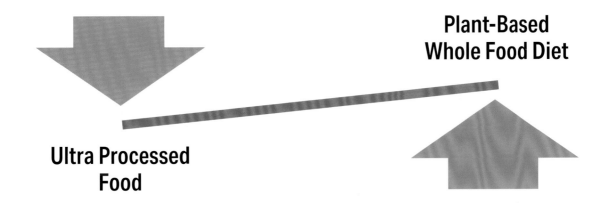

Plant-Based Whole Food Diet

Ultra Processed Food

What I'm trying to say is, it's complicated. Many scientists feel the NOVA classification system doesn't match up to other food-based classification systems. For example, on the UK's standard food labelling system a meat-free mince product might score green for fat, saturated fat and sugar, and amber for salt. But it would also be considered ultra-processed because it has more than five ingredients, many of which are necessary additives. So, should we be eating it or not? It's messy, it's a minefield, and it's confusing. Generally speaking, most people (including me, until I started researching the NOVA system for this book) find it quite difficult to place products into clear categories of processing. For example, some crisps are obviously ultra-processed, but if a brand has a crisp with only potato, salt and oil in its ingredients list, that wouldn't be as processed. Similarly, a burger from a fast-food chain will almost certainly be ultra-processed, but if you buy a fresh burger made of ground mince, egg and seasoning, is that ultra-processed? Luckily, new online apps are emerging to help people classify UPFs, and if this is something that you are now interested in, you may wish to download a couple and check out a few of your favourite foods.

UPFS AND YOU

Because of how ingrained UPFs are in our society, learning about ultra-processed foods can be confusing and may make you feel some interesting emotions when you realise quite how ultra-processed some of the 'healthy' marketed snacks are. On top of that, for many people, trying to reduce the amount of ultra-processed foods they eat can come with complications such as increased cost, breaking habits, dealing with shorter shelf lives, changing preferences and adjusting to longer preparation times.

The bottom line is that knowledge is power. The more we know, the more we can understand the potential harmful effects on our health, and the more we can make informed, balanced choices about which ultra-processed foods we choose to eat. Overall, the overwhelming evidence and consensus is that reducing our UPF intake is extremely likely to be beneficial to our overall health. However, for many of the reasons I have mentioned above, less forceful or prescriptive recommendations for UPF intake are also extremely important, and the recipes in this book have been designed with this in mind, minimising the use of UPFs without being judgemental about them.

Looking at our whole diet, rather than at individual products, is key. However, as a doctor I have looked at a lot of the scientific evidence and it's my firm belief that if, as families or individuals, you find that over half your food intake is coming from ultra-processed foods, reducing your consumption of these foods by 20 per cent or more will likely result in tangible health gains. And if you can cut down the overall contribution of UPFs to less than 10 per cent of your diet, you are likely on to a winner. Ultimately it is all about shifting that pendulum to make your diet, where possible, predominantly a plant-based whole food one.

'Plant-Forward' Your Life

Now that we have explored the far-reaching impact of a healthy gut and the benefits of increasing plant diversity and reducing ultra-processed food, it's probably time to start looking at how we might actually go about doing it.

I don't want to get preachy about any of this, but I want to share with you a life-changing positive approach to achieving your personal gut health goals that I have found to be extremely useful in changing my own food mindset. Naturally, it has had a huge impact on how my family eats as well.

This approach is self-directed and will get you focused on your eating habits in a way that you perhaps may not have done in the past. By the end of the process I hope you will feel more secure in understanding your own food relationships, and more confident when selecting the recipes from this book and identifying which of them will be of most benefit to your health. You can choose to do this exercise as a family, with your partner or on your own.

This process will obviously not be as refined as if you were to do the same exercise with a dietitian or nutritionist, but it is nonetheless still very worthwhile to try at home. For me, it provided a more focused approach than if I were to just randomly select recipes to cook here and there, which if we are honest is how most of us have interacted with recipe books in the past.

THE THREE STEPS ARE AS FOLLOWS:

- Step 1 Discover
  The first step of this process is to discover which foods you actually eat. You will carefully and honestly identify all the foods that you have eaten (either individually or as a family) in the past week and critically evaluate how much of your diet was based on plant-based whole foods versus ultra-processed food items. Remember, there is no judgement here; this is simply an information-gathering exercise.

- Step 2 Reframe
  In the next step you will carefully look at the parts of your diet where maximum gains can be made, and then make targeted 'SMART' goals for you or your whole family to focus on.

- Step 3 Realise Your Goals
  Lastly, you will look at some of the barriers you might face when it comes to achieving the goals you set, and what you can do to get around them. This is a self-reflection exercise.

This process can be a standalone exercise, or it can be a cyclical process that you revisit every few months, feeding the results of the first cycle into the new goals of the second. In time, the progress you have made with the goals you set yourself should become apparent, and you will be able to see first-hand the tangible benefits of reducing ultra-processed food consumption and increasing plant-based food intake.

STEP 1 DISCOVER

Sometimes it's pretty obvious where our diet is lacking in plant-based diversity, and other times we need to take a step back and work it out. This is a dietary information-gathering exercise and will take around 15 minutes. It can be done for each person, or for the whole family together.

Start by making a food diary of what you have eaten in the last five to seven days. You should include all snacks and drinks, no matter how small. I realise that it is hard to think back at everything you ate in the last week, and your recall may not be 100 per cent accurate but try your best to be as detailed as possible and don't forget those snack items! Here is a template for you to use.

	BREAKFAST	LUNCH	DINNER	SNACKS	DRINKS
Monday					
Tuesday					
Wednesday					
Thursday					
Friday					
Saturday					
Sunday					

ONCE YOU HAVE FILLED IN THE ABOVE, USE TWO HIGHLIGHTERS OR COLOURED PENS AS FOLLOWS:

- Highlight those items which are predominantly whole food plant-based meals with one colour (GREEN).

- Highlight those items which are clearly ultra-processed food items using the other colour (ORANGE). (*For guidance on which foods are ultra-processed, see page 17.*)

- Some items may be both ultra-processed and plant-based, for example, toasted white bread with a chickpea and tomato salad. Highlight these items half and half with both colours.

- Some items like meat, dairy and fluids may not fit into any group, so leave these un-highlighted.

- Don't worry too much if you can't place a food item in a set category, it's the overall picture that we are after here.

STEP 2 REFRAME

Now that you have had a chance to look at the components of your diet and identify which are plant-based whole foods and which are UPFs, take a step back and look at the whole picture.

KEY QUESTIONS TO ASK:

- Are any patterns emerging for you or the family as a whole?
- Are there particular times or meals where you are doing well?
- Are the ultra-processed items you eat clustered around any particular times of the day?
- Is there a lack of plant-based diversity at a particular mealtime?

Here are two worked examples for you to look at. Plant-based items are highlighted in green and UPFs are highlighted in orange.

EXAMPLE 1

Shows that there may be benefit in incorporating more plant-based foods at lunchtime and perhaps rethinking snack habits.
A good starting point would therefore be the Lunch and Snack chapters. If you only have 20 minutes of time a day to spare, this is where most health gains will be made.

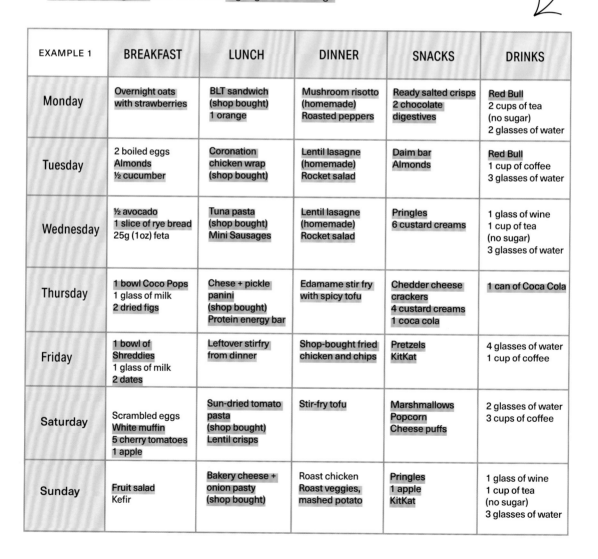

EXAMPLE 1	BREAKFAST	LUNCH	DINNER	SNACKS	DRINKS
Monday	Overnight oats with strawberries	BLT sandwich (shop bought) 1 orange	Mushroom risotto (homemade) Roasted peppers	Ready salted crisps 2 chocolate digestives	Red Bull 2 cups of tea (no sugar) 2 glasses of water
Tuesday	2 boiled eggs Almonds ½ cucumber	Coronation chicken wrap (shop bought)	Lentil lasagne (homemade) Rocket salad	Daim bar Almonds	Red Bull 1 cup of coffee 3 glasses of water
Wednesday	½ avocado 1 slice of rye bread 25g (1oz) feta	Tuna pasta (shop bought) Mini Sausages	Lentil lasagne (homemade) Rocket salad	Pringles 6 custard creams	1 glass of wine 1 cup of tea (no sugar) 3 glasses of water
Thursday	1 bowl Coco Pops 1 glass of milk 2 dried figs	Chese + pickle panini (shop bought) Protein energy bar	Edamame stir fry with spicy tofu	Chedder cheese crackers 4 custard creams 1 coca cola	1 can of Coca Cola
Friday	1 bowl of Shreddies 1 glass of milk 2 dates	Leftover stirfry from dinner	Shop-bought fried chicken and chips	Pretzels KitKat	4 glasses of water 1 cup of coffee
Saturday	Scrambled eggs White muffin 5 cherry tomatoes 1 apple	Sun-dried tomato pasta (shop bought) Lentil crisps	Stir-fry tofu	Marshmallows Popcorn Cheese puffs	2 glasses of water 3 cups of coffee
Sunday	Fruit salad Kefir	Bakery cheese + onion pasty (shop bought)	Roast chicken Roast veggies, mashed potato	Pringles 1 apple KitKat	1 glass of wine 1 cup of tea (no sugar) 3 glasses of water

Plant-Forward Your Life

EXAMPLE 2	BREAKFAST	LUNCH	DINNER	SNACKS	DRINKS
Monday	Crunchy nut cornflakes and milk	Root vegetable soup (canteen)	Beef lasagne Garden peas	Mixed nuts 1 orange Breaksticks	2 cups of coffee 2 cans of Coca Cola
Tuesday	Crunchy nut cornflakes and milk	Daal with brown rice (canteen)	Roast chicken Bulgar wheat salad	1 packet crisps Mixed nuts	2 cups of coffee 1 can of Coca Cola 1 Fanta
Wednesday	2 slices of white bread with Nutella	Skipped lunch	Fish + chips (from frozen)	Dried apricots and goji berries Seaweed crisps	3 cups of coffee 1 glass water 1 can Coca Cola
Thursday	Crunchy nut cornflakes and milk	Mushroom stroganoff with rice (canteen)	Chicken curry Wld rice Mixed salad	1 banana 1 tangerine	2 cups of coffee 1 glass of water
Friday	2 slices of white bread with crunchy peanut butter	Prawn + peanut salad	Chicken curry Wld rice Mixed salad	Mini sausages 1 apple	4 cans of Coca Cola 1 cup of tea
Saturday	Crunchy nut cornflakes and milk	Scampi + chips	Stuffed peppers with lamb mince	Mixed nuts and raisins	2 cups of coffee 1 can of Coca Cola 1 Fanta
Sunday	2 slices of white bread with Nutella	Skipped lunch	Roast beef Horseradish sauce (homemade) Garden peas		3 cups of coffee 1 can of Coca Cola

EXAMPLE 2

Identifies a diet where the breakfast options have become monotonous, and where attention should be given to drinking more water and improving overall hydration. Perhaps fizzy sweetened beverages could be substituted for a probiotic kombucha? If changes are to be made, breakfast would be a good starting point, so the Breakfast and Brunch chapters will hopefully be of interest to this person. As another separate observation, there is heavy a reliance on meat and poultry items at dinner time, which could be substituted for plant-based alternatives from the Dinner chapter.

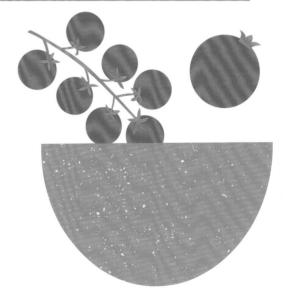

Now that you have discovered the reality of your eating habits, it's time to use this newfound knowledge about yours and your family's diet. It's time to generate a **SMART** goal. This is an acronym we use quite a lot across the medical field, and I find it a helpful tool to set clear, meaningful and attainable targets. **SMART** goals must be:

1. SPECIFIC
   What exactly do you want to accomplish? Exactly what will you do and why is it important?

2. MEASURABLE
   How will you know whether you have met the goal? Is there a way of keeping an eye on how things are progressing? Quantify your goals if possible.

3. ACHIEVABLE
   Is the goal realistic? Do you have the skills and resources at your disposal to make the goal a reality? The goal should stretch you a little but still remain attainable.

4. RELEVANT
   How and why is this goal worthwhile? Does this goal line up with others around you? Is it the right time and will it improve your life?

5. TIMEBOUND
   Have you set yourself a deadline for achieving the goal?

For example, one of your goals might be to 'make more of the family's lunches at home'. Here is a real-life example of how the SMART approach to goal-setting works.

SPECIFIC: 'This goal is specific to our needs as a family. We have identified that we are buying far too many ultra-processed, expensive lunches from the shops, so it makes sense to batch-cook some lunch options in advance. We have had a look at some of the portable lunch options together in this book and plan on using them as a starting point.'

MEASURABLE: 'We will keep a diary of how many home-made lunchboxes we manage to make per week. We will put a small tick next to the days of the week where we manage to meet our goal. If we get time, we will also list the recipes that we all really liked.'

ACHIEVABLE: 'It might be difficult for us to achieve this change all at once, so we will try to batch-cook our lunch once a week to start with, and then will increase this to two or three times a week over the next month or so. We already have enough Tupperware containers and plenty of fridge space, as long as we just re-organise some of the jars that are taking up extra space. My partner and I will do the majority of the lunch preparation for the family. The children can participate in the washing up if the parents do the cooking!'

RELEVANT: 'People around us are also trying to do the same, particularly at school and at our workplaces. We will have a chat with the people who bring their own lunch from home about what lunch options they have and try and build more of a lunch community instead of eating alone. This is a worthwhile goal for us as we can use lunch as an opportunity to increase fibre intake and regularise our bowel habits. We have been prone to constipation as a family, and this has been an even bigger issue recently when we don't manage to get enough fibre.'

TIMEBOUND: 'We really want to make this an indefinite change but understand that we will have to ease ourselves into it. We will start by setting a three-month target and seeing how far we have come at this point. We want to see an improvement from Day 0 to Day 90, and even if we haven't achieved perfection, we will not be hard on ourselves.'

I'll admit, at first glance the SMART approach does sound a bit over the top, and it might feel a little forced when you write out your first few SMART targets. But honestly, this approach is one of the best ways I know to focus on your goals. It's far from the predictable New Year's Resolution you set yourself that you subsequently forgot by mid-January; this is a quantifiable, measurable, accountable target that will propel you to the action plan stage and will pay dividends on your gut-health journey.

STEP 3 REALISE YOUR GOALS

Here we take a look at the challenges you and your family might face when trying to hit your nutrition goals. Eating is a behaviour and as a doctor I can tell you that changing health-related behaviours can be exceptionally, painfully hard. Whether that means changing what you eat, stopping smoking, or prioritising exercise and sleep, it is not an easy task.

Health psychologists have come up with a variety of models to understand how and whether people will change certain behaviours. One such model is the 'COMB' model and was developed by Professor Susan Michie at University College London. This is the Rolls-Royce of behaviour models; at the time of writing, her paper explaining the model has been cited by over 10,000 scientific papers.

Michie's model states that any health behaviour, be it eating more plant-based foods or cutting down on ultra-processed snacks, is an interaction between three necessary conditions: **Capability, Opportunity and Motivation** – only then can you change **Behaviour**. Now that you have set your **SMART** goals, it's time to think about your own/ your family's capability, motivation and opportunity, to give yourself the best chance to reach the health goals you have set. I have simplified the model a little for ease here, but you can look at the individual components in more detail if you wish.

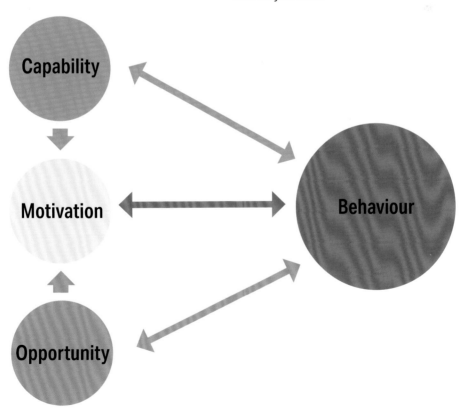

Capability

This assesses whether you have both the physical and psychological ability to eat a gut-healthy diet.

- **How confident are you at cooking?** *A student leaving home for the first time may need to improve their basic cookery skills before they feel ready to face the kitchen without anxiety.*
- **What sort of physical space do you have to cook in?** *A family kitchen that is very small, cluttered or lacks equipment can make cooking difficult.*
- **How good is your knowledge about gut-healthy eating?** *Do all family members feel confident identifying gut-healthy food items when shopping?*
- **How often are you able to take a step back to think about your diet?** *A busy or stressed person just might not have the head space to think about food.*

Opportunity

This refers to whether you are in an environment that enables you to eat gut-healthy food as a family/individual.

- **How you are going to afford the ingredients necessary to achieve your health goals?** *Someone who has recently had a pay cut or mortgage rise will have to carefully assess which recipes are most cost-effective.*
- **Do you have any time to cook?** *Someone who works night shifts might struggle to work out when to cook for the family. It might need to be carefully scheduled into the diary. Mothers of young children will also have to work around their children's needs.*
- **How easy is it to get the ingredients you need?** *Some people don't have a car to drive to their local supermarket and all the local food shops are fast-food outlets. How will they make sure their fridge and cupboards are stocked with the food they need?*
- **To what extent will your family and friends be an active part of the dietary change you are going to make?** *If your partner is really not keen on the food that you will be cooking, is this going to influence your likelihood of achieving your health goals?*

Motivation

This refers to the conscious and unconscious internal thought processes that influence whether we choose a gut-healthy diet or not.

- **How easy or difficult do you think it will be to reduce your intake of ultra-processed foods?**
- **How confident do you feel about overcoming some of the challenges you will face when changing the way you eat?** *A person's confidence may have taken a knock in the past where they have tried hard to make dietary changes, but they haven't managed to sustain change.*
- **Would eating a gut-healthy diet make you feel happy and healthy?** *Does the person truly believe that this pattern of eating will benefit their health in the short and long term?*
- **Are there other fears or emotions that have held you back?** *The mental processes behind eating can be extremely complicated. Those who have had periods of disordered or restrictive eating may find making changes in their diet very triggering, and this could even signal a need for further help in this situation.*

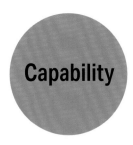

Capability

I know about this.
I can do this.

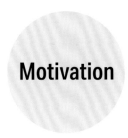

Motivation

I feel I want to do this.

I believe this is the right thing to do.

I have the right habits in place.

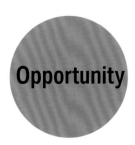

Opportunity

I have what I need to
do this.

Other approve of me
doing this.

By thinking your way through this behaviour change model in a structured way, it is my hope that you can understand more fully the factors that are key to you changing some of your personal and/or your family's eating behaviours. After around 4 to 8 weeks of following this method, have another go at the reframing exercise on page 24 – this is often a really rewarding exercise and you may find that you have made significant changes. In addition, have a think about whether you need to tweak any of your SMART goals. Remember, the whole process is a marathon, not a sprint. Some ups and downs are expected as you navigate the tricky business of changing your eating habits to include more gut-healthy foods.

I hope that by going through this self-reflection process, you will be more able to sustain any positive changes to your eating habits that you identify, and that you can improve your gut health while also enjoying an array of super practical, nutritious, and delicious, 20-minute recipes.

There are no calorie counts listed for my recipes and this is completely intentional. The calorie, although useful in some circumstances, is really a blunt instrument when it comes to nutritional science. Restriction of calories is a source of stress and anxiety for so many people I meet and I'd much prefer for you to concentrate on diversity in the foods that make up your diet rather than focus on calorie restriction. Each recipe contains not just a diversity count, but also tips on how to achieve extra diversity points for those looking to go that extra mile. The fibre content per portion is also listed, which I hope will help you achieve your 30g of fibre a day target.

How to Shop

The vast majority of the ingredients required for these recipes are easily found in mainstream supermarkets, so shopping for them should not be a challenge. What's more, the recipes in this book have a strong reliance on store cupboard and freezer ingredients, with an emphasis on fruits, vegetables and whole grains. Ultra-processed food items are used as little as possible while fermented foods are used generously throughout.

These are my top tips for making your weekly shop as stress free as possible. Remember shopping for food can be a source of pleasure, rather than an activity that provokes anxiety.

TIP 1:
ADVANCE PLANNING

If you can have even a rough meal plan ready for the week ahead, it will focus your shopping and will hopefully lead to less food wastage. We are all too familiar with the fruit and vegetables bought with the best of intentions that instead end up going off at the back of the fridge because we never got a chance to get around to them. Instead get into the habit of buying, cooking and eating with intention. Planning meals with the people you live with is particularly beneficial. Children often engage very well when they have had a say in what will be cooked! Encourage your kids or partner to flick through the pages of this book and flagging up dishes they want to try.

TIP 2:
DON'T SHOP WHEN YOU'RE HUNGRY

There is compelling data that suggests that the contents of our shopping trolleys differ depending on whether we shop with a full stomach or an empty one. We've all been there; there's nothing worse than coming back from your weekly shop to find that you forgot the bread, milk and eggs but somehow came home with three packs of biscuits and a variety pack of crisps.

TIP 3:
TAKE TIME TO LOOK AT INGREDIENTS LISTS FOR COMMON FOOD ITEMS

Food items like bread and yoghurt often have very long ingredients lists and if they have added preservatives, emulsifiers, sweeteners etc., they are likely to be ultra-processed. If you familiarise yourself with the ingredients lists you will quickly be able to identify which products are less processed and can then safely add these to your trolley every time your shop.

TIP 4:
SPEND MORE OF YOUR TIME IN THESE KEY PARTS OF THE SUPERMARKET

- **Zone 1:** Fresh fruit and vegetables. I always eyeball which vegetables are on special offer on the day and assess if there is potential to bulk buy and freeze.

- **Zone 2:** Tinned lentils, chickpeas and other pulses, dried whole grains and vacuum-packed pre-cooked grains.

- **Zone 3:** Nuts and spices – these are often particularly good value when bought in the World Foods section.

- **Zone 4:** Frozen ingredients e.g. peas, carrots, cauliflower, spinach, onions and mixed fruits of every assortment.

TIP 5:
FACTOR IN A TREAT

Once you have filled your trolley from zones 1–4 of the supermarket, allow yourself one or two items from the snack zone. For me, this is Bombay mix, for you it might be a sausage roll or a bar of chocolate. Life's too short to completely miss out on these simple but wonderful pleasures.

Practical Tips for Success in 20 Minutes

ORGANISE YOUR KITCHEN SPACE

I can't stress enough how important an organised kitchen is to the success of your gut-health journey. All my cookery books have been written in my cramped west London kitchen. There's hardly enough space for two people to stand, but as it's the only way to get from the house to the garden it's also a busy thoroughfare. But with a bit of planning, I've managed to turn what could be a hellish kitchenscape into an area of relative calm. Here are a few pointers to make even the smallest of spaces work for you.

Firstly, decluttering your work surface is essential. Nothing is left on the work surface except for my toaster, kettle and a small air fryer. I have a space designated to my chopping board and this is where the majority of food preparation happens.

I have a cupboard next to the cooker where I tuck away my food processor and blender so that they are easily 'grabbable' when needed. Sometimes, if I know I need my blender for breakfast the next morning, I leave it ready on the work surface for use first thing in the morning. Overall, the less cluttered your work surfaces are, generally the easier it will be for you to function in a small kitchen space, and the clearer and calmer your mind will be while you cook.

Secondly, I don't advocate using lots of fancy equipment in the kitchen. I very much don't feel that any of us need to have a slow cooker and a bread maker and an ice cream maker out on the kitchen counter 24/7. I'll always recommend you invest in good-quality Tupperware or glass sealable boxes, especially if you plan on batch-cooking or doing packed lunches for yourself. In my experience, this is one of those times when paying a bit more for a good brand can be an excellent decision. Remember, you won't think about that fiver you saved getting the cheaper Tupperware box when it opens in your bag and spills your lunch on to your laptop.

These are the key pieces of kitchen equipment I recommend and you'll notice that the recipes in this book rely heavily on this equipment to save precious time. They make great birthday presents too.

A NOTE ON AIR FRYERS

For many years we have relied on just the hob, oven, grill and microwave to cook our food. Then along comes the air fryer, a device that helps achieve the results of an oven/grill in a mere fraction of the time and at a lesser energy cost overall. This gadget appeals to my lazy side in a way that no other culinary instrument really can and sadly, a microwave can simply never achieve the same textural result. You can get the most glorious charred finish to vegetables and meat dishes in the air fryer and I have used the air fryer in a few of these recipes to hit the 20-minute target. However, if you don't have air fryer, an alternative oven/grill cookery method is provided.

Key pieces of Kitchen Kit

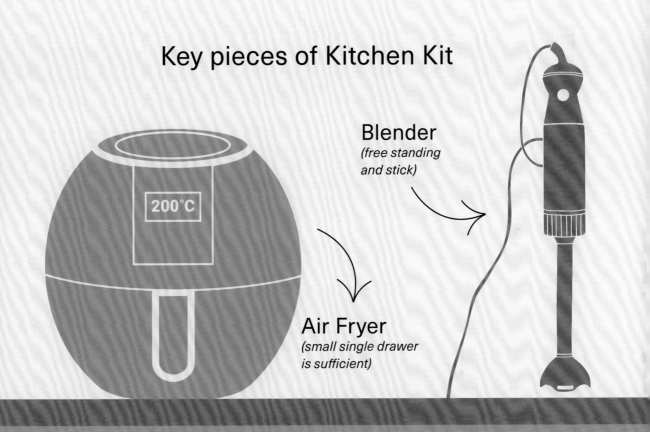

Blender
(free standing and stick)

200°C

Air Fryer
(small single drawer is sufficient)

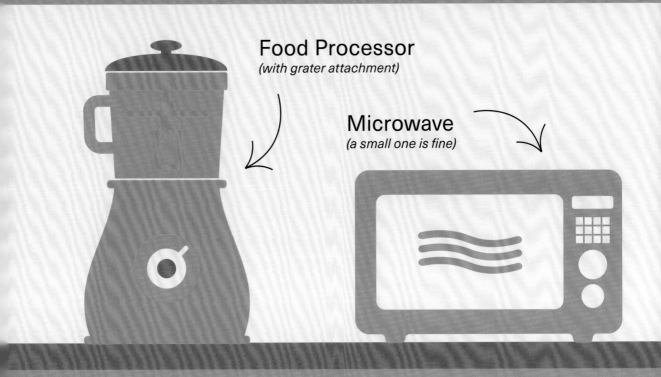

Food Processor
(with grater attachment)

Microwave
(a small one is fine)

STOCK UP YOUR FLAVOUR CABINET

On busy weekday evenings most of us simply don't have time to chop onions, peel garlic, slice ginger and make fancy spice pastes. Luckily, there are shortcuts for almost all these basic ingredients that will, over the course of a year, save you literally entire days in prep time.

Instead of peeling and chopping onions, why not buy frozen chopped onions from the freezer section and just grab what you need to chuck into a pan whenever you need it? Garlic can be bought peeled, chopped and frozen, or in paste form, as can ginger, saving you the trouble of peeling and chopping it yourself.

When it comes to stocking up my 'flavour' cabinet, you'll always find the following in my kitchen. I simply can't get by without these flavour bombs. They are well worth stocking up on as they are relatively inexpensive and have long shelf lives.

Spice mixes
- Peri peri rub
- Shawarma seasoning
- Za'atar
- Ras el hanout or baharat spice mix
- Curry powder
- Garam masala

Flavour jars
- Harissa paste
- Chipotle paste
- Soy sauce
- Miso paste
- Chiu Chow chilli oil
- Crispy chillies in oil (I like Lao Gan Ma brand)
- Garlic paste
- Ginger paste
- Lemongrass paste
- Gochujang paste
- Sun-dried tomatoes
- Jarred peppers
- Jalfrezi and/or korma paste
- Thai green curry paste
- Peanut butter

SUNDAY NIGHTS

Earlier, I touched upon the importance of meal planning. For me it's all about Sunday nights; this is the time when I organise my week, not just the ironing or the children's school uniforms, but in the kitchen too. One trick I find helpful is to prep or pre-cook any carbohydrates I want to eat over the next few days and have them ready in the fridge. For example, one week I might boil and drain some quinoa before cooling and refrigerating. Another week it might be bulgur wheat, brown rice or pearl barley instead. And if you are using dried lentils instead of tinned, you can pre-cook these too. The greater the variety, the better. That said, I often rely on those vacuum-packed pouches of pre-cooked grains and pulses – brands like Merchant Gourmet have been a saviour. I thoroughly recommend their use if you don't have the time, or you just can't bring yourself to prepare your starches on a Sunday!

While the grains are bubbling away, I might also pop the oven on and roast some sweet potatoes, parsnips, carrots or beetroot, depending on my mood and what's in my fridge.

When you have these food items sitting ready in the fridge, it becomes really easy to bring them out for lunch or dinner; all you need to do is add some fresh produce, a few store cupboard ingredients, perhaps some spices and any herbs you have to hand. The other benefit of cooking and then cooling vegetables in this way means that they develop 'resistant starches' on their surface, which are felt to be helpful to our gut microbes.

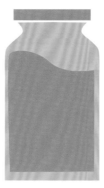
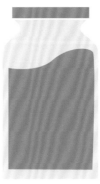
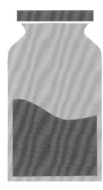

This book...

Is not a book about 'slimming' in the conventional sense, although many people will notice weight loss as a result of beneficial changes in their eating pattern. It does not promote any particular fad. I don't ask readers to drink apple cider vinegar every day or eat probiotic cookies, or any 'elixir' that is designed to 'cleanse' my insides. It is not part of a diet of exclusion. In fact, I have tried to go in the opposite direction and include as varied a macro and micro nutrient profile across recipes as possible. No complete sacrifice of food groups is expected. And finally, it does not ascribe to any 'ritualistic' pattern of eating, like intermittent fasting. The one thing I will say is that studies suggest that some regularity in when you choose to eat your meals is beneficial, in order to help regulate your body's natural circadian rhythms.

For anybody with gastrointestinal symptoms, talk to a healthcare professional about your concerns before you make any dietary changes. Working with a healthcare professional to get to the root cause of your problem is a better approach than reliance on quick fixes.
We live in the most confusing of food climates. Our digital lifestyles constantly bombard us with flashy headlines. Clickbait endlessly pops up, promoting extreme or simplified approaches to eating that are so far removed from the nuances of nutritional science. #Guttok may have 750 million views, but that doesn't mean that it's a credible place to find health advice. It is getting progressively harder to discern spurious gut-health trends from medical and nutritional reality.

While I was researching the 'express' recipes for this book, I quickly came to realise that many quick and easy recipes, particularly those found on platforms like TikTok, can be detrimental to our relationship with food. They promise the world, but fail to deliver on flavour, leaving many who invest time and money in making the recipes bitterly disappointed, and less willing to try other recipes. I have taken great time to make sure that flavour is never compromised in this book, and I am certain you will like the results!

Coming up with a selection of recipes that you could have on the table in 20 minutes or less was important for me but, obviously, if you find yourself taking a bit longer, don't sweat! This book is all about showing you what is possible, and I've worked out all the tips and tricks so you don't have to. I have purposefully written recipes where you don't have to rely too heavily on measuring scales and jugs. I work in teaspoons, tablespoons and handfuls. I have looked at the quantities of common packets of ingredients and tried to use all or half of the pack so that you don't waste time measuring and can work by eye as much as possible.

A final word from me: A healthy sustainable relationship with food does not start with demonising particular food groups. It does not start with being shamed for so much as looking at a chocolate bar. Healthy food relationships are built on the knowledge to make informed choices, and in realising that what counts isn't the chocolate bar you eat once a week, but the overall pattern of your diet and the diversity it contains. Before you enter your kitchen remember this: eat for pleasure, always. The sheer joy that food brings should never be forgotten.

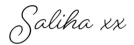

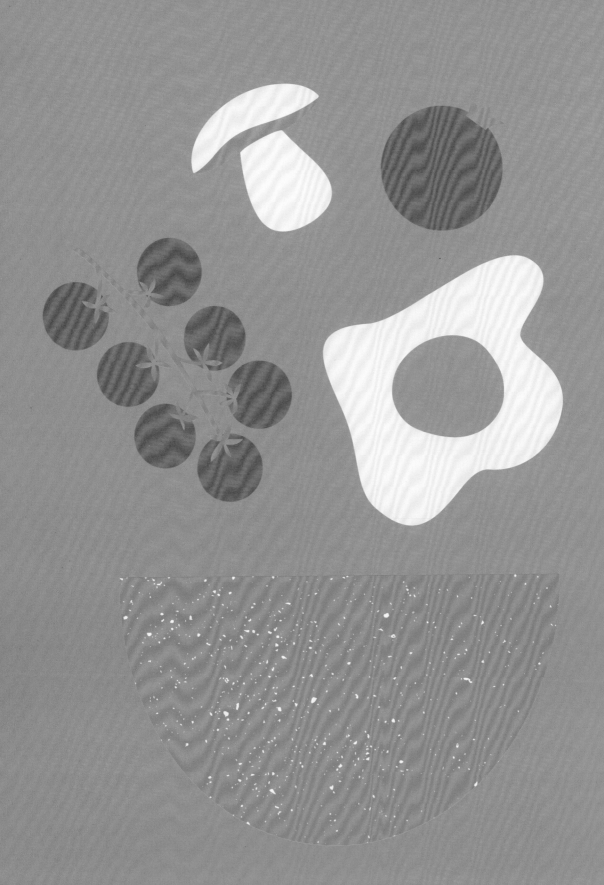

Ready
Steady
Breakfast

chapter one

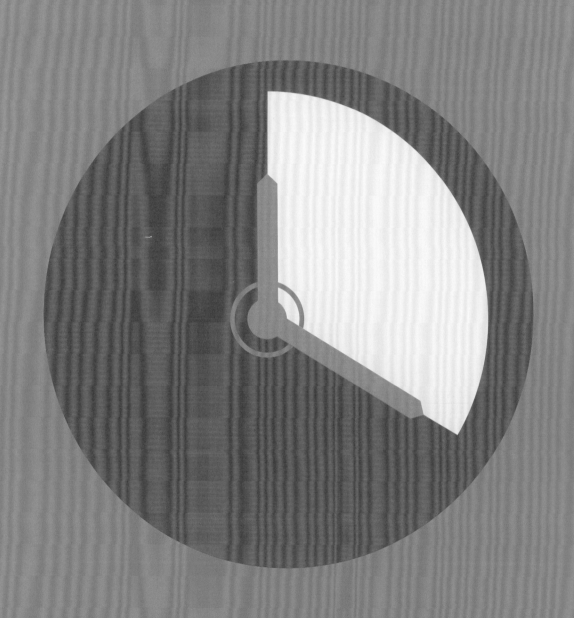

These days, there are very few mornings where I don't feel like I have woken up inside a pressure cooker, and I imagine many of you reading this feel the same way. From the moment we open our eyes we are forced into action, trying our best to get ourselves and any dependents out the door cleaned, clothed and – if we are lucky – fed.

Fitting any breakfast into our hectic lives, let alone one that requires preparation, can feel like an impossible dream, which is why it's often one of the first things to fall by the wayside in our battle to get out of the house. But does it have to be like this?

In this chapter I want to share some simple but tasty breakfast ideas that you can make before bedtime the night before, ready for you to grab and go in the morning, plus some other recipes that are quick enough to pull together in the morning while still leaving you with plenty of time to hunt for your coffee cup, jacket and keys.

My goal with these recipes is to move breakfast away from the realm of beige cereal and give it a good shove towards a landscape of colour, texture, nutrition and joy. I'm also hoping that these recipes will show you how easy it can be to break away from the idea of a 'good' breakfast being a 45-minute stovetop ordeal that somehow dirties every pan you own.

However, before we go into these new breakfast recipes in more detail, there are a couple of questions worth asking. For me, these are: what is your relationship with breakfast? And are you making the most of this precious mealtime? I have lost count of the number of people I meet who miss breakfast and then get so hungry by mid-morning that they snack on whatever they can find in the vending machine, or end up consuming a humungous lunch at the first opportunity. This isn't surprising: when our bodies feel like they are starving, they do what they are designed to do. They find a rapid energy source, they consume calories, they survive.

It is therefore clear to me that *what* you eat for breakfast is far more important than whether or not you eat breakfast. My view is simple: have breakfast if you like breakfast, but if you're going to do it, do it better! Why limit yourself to cereal and toast on repeat if tastier, healthier and equally convenient options exist?

Through the recipes in this chapter, I'll show you how to work towards increasing the diversity of plant-based foods that you eat, right from the start of the day. We will also feature glorious probiotics, like kefir and live yoghurt. Lastly, given the sheer number of great breakfast options that are naturally dense in fibre (oats, nuts, seeds and fruit), these recipes will set your gut up for a great day by increasing your fibre intake from the get-go.

Breakfast can, if done right, be the first act of self-care we perform in our day; a commitment to looking after ourselves. I hope that these recipes make a difference to your mornings, and that they provide some enjoyable alternatives to the usual pastries that we all grab so often.

Super Speedy Breakfast Banana Split

Diversity points: 7 / Fibre: 10g

1 medium sized ripe banana

100g (3½oz) full-fat live Greek yoghurt, or labneh

2 dried figs

1 Palestinian Medjool date

1 tbsp peanuts

1 tbsp pecan nuts

1 tbsp toasted pumpkin seeds

1 tbsp date molasses or 1 teaspoon honey

1 tbsp tahini paste or any runny nut butter

A few curls of dark chocolate (optional)

+ Bonus Diversity Points
1 tablespoon toasted coconut, a handful of blueberries and ½ teaspoon cinnamon powder can be sprinkled over the top of the banana split if you wish.

I was inspired by this recipe when my little one asked for ice cream for breakfast. He wanted banana split, so I delivered! Feel free to top the banana split with any berries that you have lying around in the fridge. It is a very flexible recipe, but really cold, live (probiotic) full fat Greek yoghurt is essential.

1. Peel the banana and discard the skin. Slice the banana in half lengthways, placing it on your plate, just as you would with a banana split.

2. Place the yoghurt in a large scoop in the centre of the banana.

3. Remove the seed from the date and chop it roughly with the dried figs. Scatter the dates and figs over the yoghurt along with the peanuts, pecans and toasted pumpkin seeds. You can chop the nuts if you wish, but I often just leave them whole to save time.

4. To complete the dish drizzle over the date molasses, tahini and dark chocolate curls.

 ## Time Saving Hacks
Instead of using individual nuts and seeds and portioning them out, use a pre mixed bag. Have your dried fruits and nuts in jars on your worktop counter so that you can grab them easily at breakfast time.

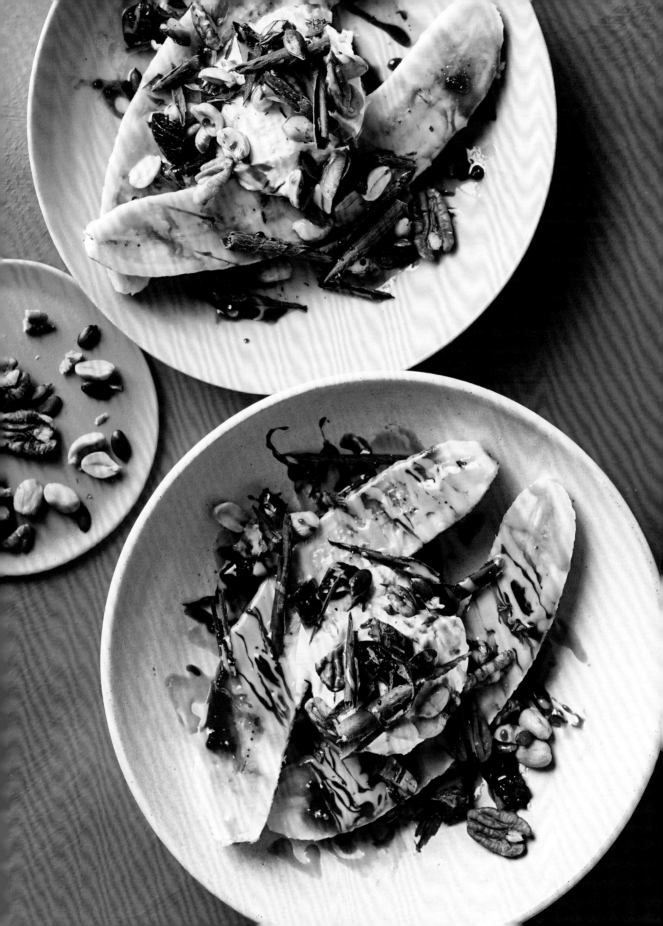

Cottage Cheese + Yummy Things on Toast

Nectarines, Honey + Chilli

Diversity points: 2 / Fibre: 12g

1 small nectarine, stoned and finely sliced
1 tsp chilli oil
1 tsp roughly chopped pistachios
1 tsp maple syrup or honey (optional)

Roasted Jar Peppers, Pomegranate + Tomatoes

Diversity points: 3. Fibre: 11g

50g jarred peppers in olive oil
3 cherry tomatoes halved
1 tbsp pomegranate seeds
½ tsp dried oregano

Crisp Pear, Walnuts, Sesame + Honey

Diversity points: 3. Fibre: 13g

½ pear sliced finely
4 walnuts roughly chopped/ broken by hand
1 tsp tahini paste
1 tsp honey (optional)
1 tsp sesame seeds (black/ white or mix)

Cottage cheese is having a bit of a revolution these days, and for good reason. It is a wonderfully filling, protein rich cheese which has long been neglected. I used to feel rather un-trendy picking it up every week, but gladly those days are behind us.

Cottage cheese does beg for the addition of intense flavour, hence the toast ideas below. This recipe really is a blueprint, and you can use any of the delicious detritus lurking at the back of your fridge to avoid food wastage.

2 small, thick slices of wholemeal sourdough bread or one large thick slice of sourdough
3 tablespoons plain, full fat unflavoured cottage cheese
Salt, to taste

1. Toast your bread in the toaster or in a frying pan on the stove top. Try to get the bread to a deep, golden brown colour. Top the toasted bread with cottage cheese, followed by the toppings listed. Season with a little salt to taste. Serve immediately.

+ Bonus Diversity Points
for a treat, try other seedy, unprocessed breads, like rye bread, Ezekiel, pumpernickel, spelt or buckwheat loaves.

Time Saving Hack
Ask the baker to slice your sourdough loaf for you so you don't have to spend time cutting even slices and spreading crumbs all over the work surface.

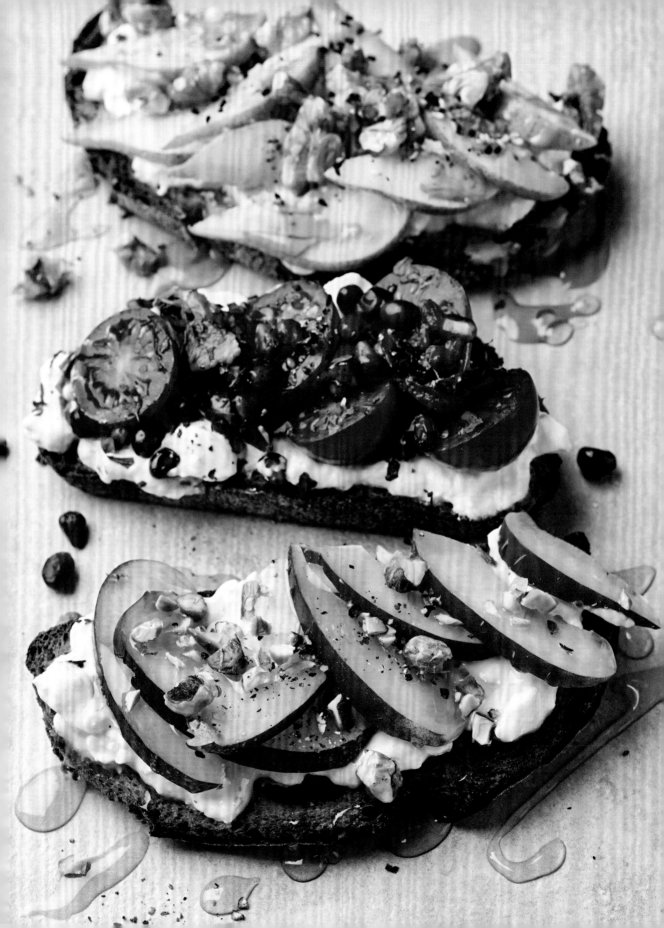

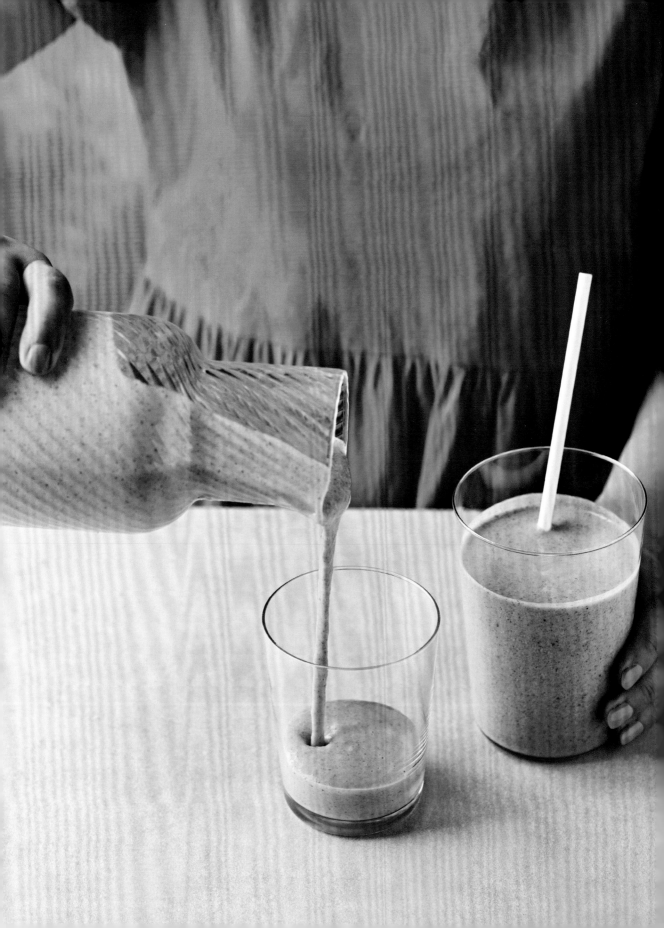

Queen of Kefir Green Smoothie

Diversity points: 5 / Fibre: 4.4g

1kg (2lb 4oz) Polish kefir (Yeo Valley and Biotiful also work well)

2 frozen bananas

4 large handfuls of frozen spinach leaves (or use frozen kale)

100g (3½oz) frozen mango

100g (3½oz) frozen pineapple

4 tbsp flaxseeds

+ Bonus Diversity Points
1 tablespoon oats, ½ avocado, ½ cucumber or a handful mint leaves can all be added to the smoothie.

Kefir is the Queen of breakfast items. I have it often – on my granola, with my oats and in my smoothies. This smoothie is light and fruity so that you can still taste the lactic, fermented probiotic tang of the kefir through it. Flaxseeds are a wonderful addition, providing both fibre and protein, and spinach leaves give it the most beautiful pastel green bucolic hue.

1. Place half the kefir into a blender with all the remaining ingredients and blitz to a smooth purée.

2. Pour the mixture out equally into two glasses and top up with the remaining kefir. Stir well and serve.

 ### Time Saving Hack
I usually have the frozen fruit and veg portioned and ready in a bag in the freezer so I can whizz up this smoothie quickly first thing in the morning. Getting the blender out on to the worktop the night before means I am ready to go!

Stovetop Chai Spiced Tahini Granola

Diversity points: 7 / Fibre: 9.6g

200g (7oz/2 cups) jumbo oats

1 heaped tbsp tahini

2 generous tbsp extra-virgin olive oil

4 tbsp maple syrup

½ tsp ground cinnamon

½ tsp ground ginger

½ tsp ground nutmeg

50g (2oz/½ cup) pecans

50g (2oz/½ cup) almonds

50g (2oz/½ cup) walnuts

50g (2oz/½ cup) hazelnuts

+ Bonus Diversity Points

Serve with some fresh or frozen fruit, a tablespoon of chia or flax seeds and probiotic yoghurt or kefir.

Granola, but no need to turn the oven on; all you need is a large, ideally non-stick frying pan. It's really lovely to make this the night before so it's ready for use and it will last a few days in an airtight jar. Try topping with live yoghurt or kefir for an extra probiotic boost.

1. Mix the oats, tahini, olive oil, maple syrup and spices together in a bowl.

2. Place a large, wide non-stick frying pan over a medium heat. Add the oats to the pan and toast for about 5 minutes, or until the oats start to turn a light golden colour. Keep stirring so that the mixture does not catch.

3. Roughly chop the nuts and drop them into the frying pan with the toasted, spiced oats. The nuts need just a minute or two more cooking. Take the pan off the heat and empty the granola on to a tray lined with baking paper. This will allow the granola to cool quickly and remain crunchy.

Time Saving Hack

If you want to save time measuring all the individual spices, why not use a spice mix like baharat or ras el hanout? Instead of measuring individual quantities of nuts, use a pre-mixed bag. Rather than wait for the granola to cool, make the granola in the morning and serve it warm with cold kefir poured over the top for contrast.

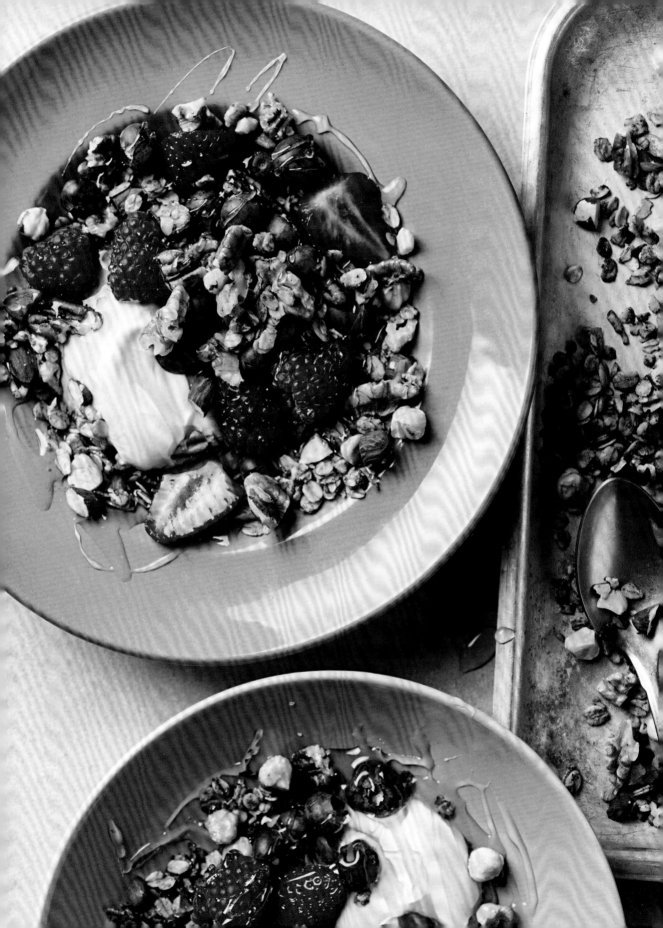

Five-Minute Overnight Oats

For the base recipe

Fibre: 5g

100g (3½oz/1 cup) jumbo oats
200ml (7fl oz/generous ¾ cup) milk of your choice
1 tbsp flaxseeds
½ tbsp chia seeds
1 tbsp full-fat live Greek yoghurt
Squeeze of honey or maple syrup (optional)
Pinch of salt (optional)

The most attractive feature of overnight oats is their endless versatility. Once you have made these a few times, you will be able to do them by eye without any measuring equipment. Here are a few of my favourite combinations. I would go as far as saying that there is an overnight oat recipe for every personality and predilection. I will let you decide what these recipes say about me.

1. Combine all the ingredients for the base recipe in a bowl and mix well to combine.

2. If you are making flavoured oats, just add all the listed ingredients from your chosen flavour combination to the base recipe and mix to combine.

3. Leave the mixture in a Tupperware box or jar in the fridge overnight to thicken. Serve cold from the fridge.

For Carrot Cake Oats

Diversity points: 7
Fibre: 5g

1 carrot, grated

½ tsp ground cinnamon

¼ tsp grated nutmeg

1 tbsp raisins

50g (2oz) roughly chopped walnuts (about a handful)

For Nutty Oats

Diversity points: 6
Fibre: 5g

50g (2oz) walnuts

50g (2oz) hazelnuts or Brazil nuts

1 tbsp crunchy peanut (or other nut) butter (palm oil free)

For Mango Lassi Oats

Diversity points: 5
Fibre: 5g

200g (7oz) small mango chunks (tinned is fine)

½ tsp fennel seeds

Seeds of 1 cardamom pod

For Black Forest Oats

Diversity points: 5
Fibre: 5g

1 tbsp cocoa powder

100g (3½oz) frozen forest fruit mixture (with at least 2 varieties of fruit)

Few curls of dark chocolate, to garnish (optional)

For Peach Melba Oats

Diversity points: 5
Fibre: 5g

50g (2oz) raspberries

½ x 400g (14oz) tin peach slices in juice (not syrup)

1 tbsp freeze-dried raspberries, to garnish (optional)

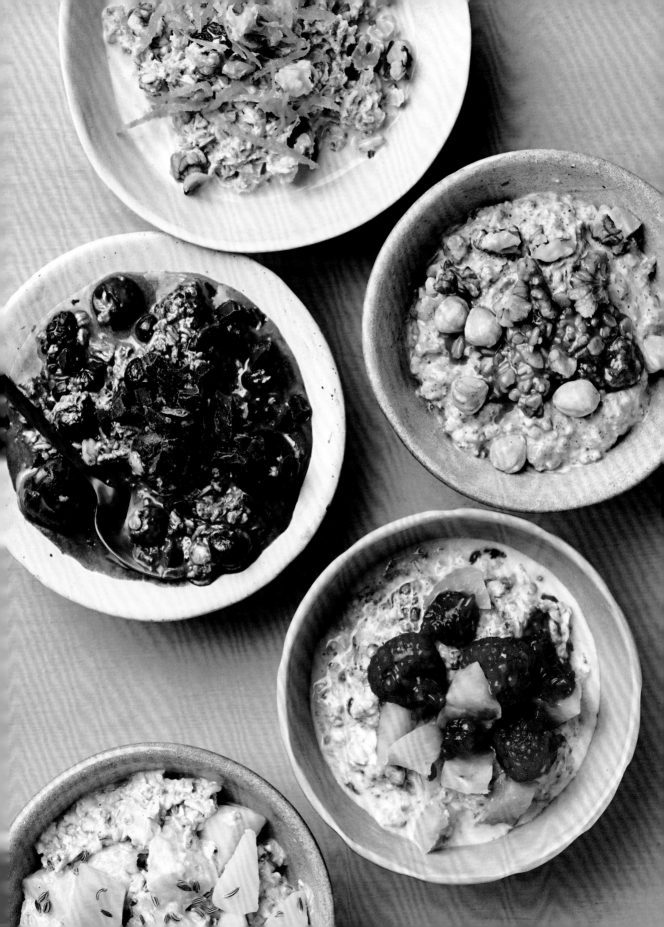

Watermelon + Blueberry Breakfast Salad

Diversity points: 5 / Fibre: 4.5g

500g (1lb 2oz) watermelon, cut into chunky cubes

125g (4oz) blueberries

1 tsp lemongrass paste

Juice of 1 lime

1 tbsp extra-virgin olive oil

1 tbsp chia seeds

Handful of basil leaves, torn (optional)

4 tbsp pumpkin seeds (optional, for crunch)

+ Bonus Diversity Points
Reduce the amount of watermelon and replace with some raspberries, kiwis or even tinned lychees in juice.

Lemongrass paste was a total game changer for me. It is found in the spice aisles of the supermarket and is usually used in savoury Thai cooking. Here in a fruit salad with lime juice it creates an explosion of unexpected flavour. Especially beautiful in the summer months where the desire for light, cool breakfasts predominates.

1. Put the watermelon and blueberries into a large, wide serving bowl.

2. In a separate small bowl, combine the lemongrass paste, lime juice and olive oil, stirring well. Drizzle this dressing over the fruit and then sprinkle over the chia seeds. Stir everything well to combine. Top with basil leaves and pumpkin seeds (if using).

Time Saving Hack
Prepare the watermelon the night before by cutting into chunks and refrigerating. Prepare the lemongrass, lime and olive oil dressing the night before and have it ready to go in a small Tupperware container.

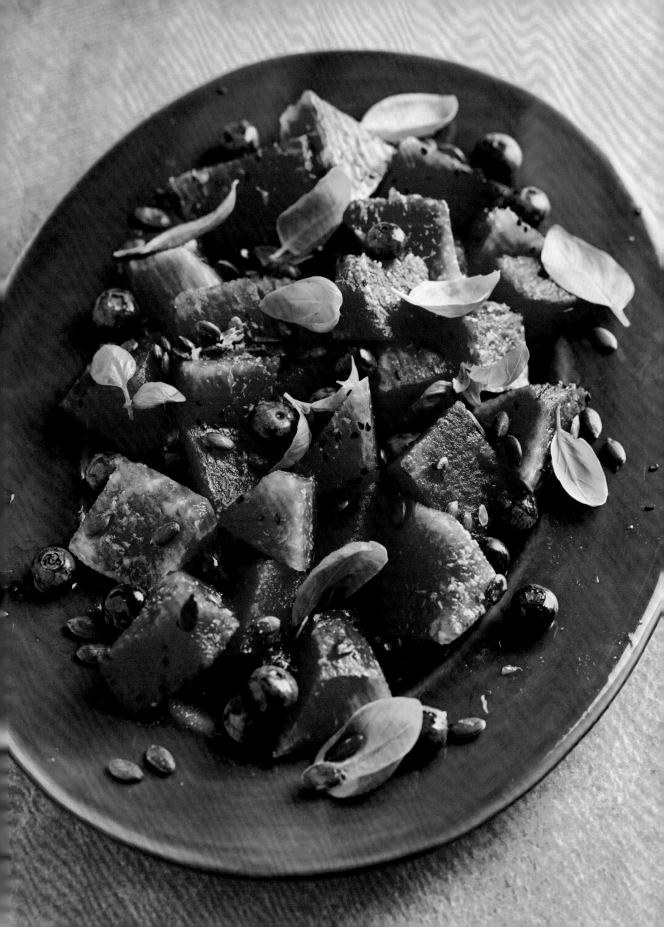

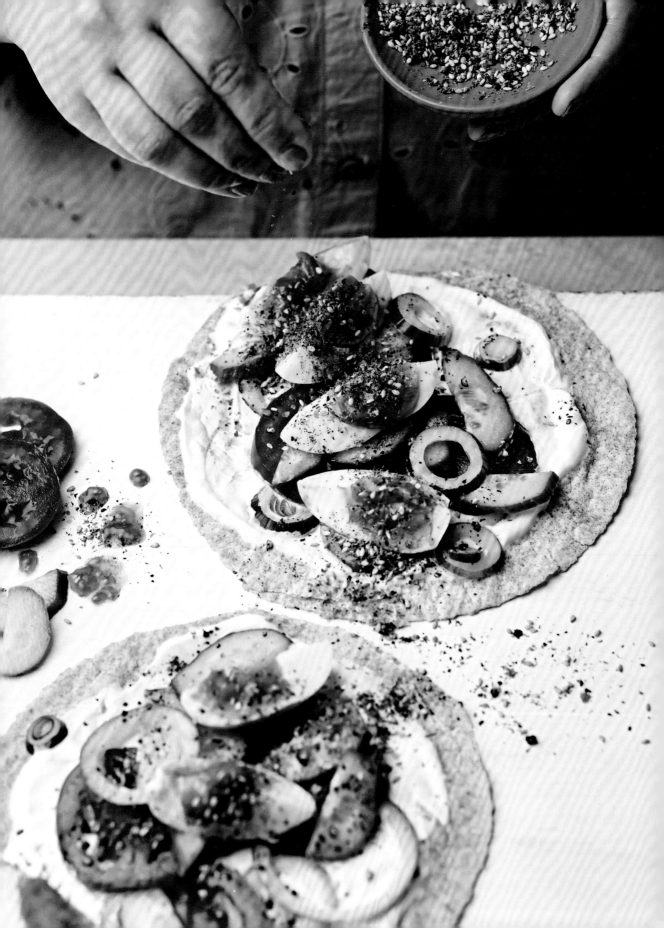

Runny Egg, Salad + Za'atar Breakfast Wraps

Diversity points: 4 / Fibre: 3.4g

2 eggs

1 lavash flatbread (30cm/12in diameter) or other pre-made wrap (I like Crosta & Mollica)

1 generous tbsp full-fat live Greek yoghurt or labneh

8cm (3in) piece of cucumber, sliced into half-moons

½ tomato, sliced

¼ red onion, thinly sliced

1 heaped tsp za'atar

Salt, to taste

+ Bonus Diversity Points
Add any of the following: 1 teaspoon capers, 1 tablespoon chickpeas, a handful of baby spinach leaves, a handful of roughly torn parsley leaves.

I am often found leaving the house with one of these wraps in hand. I find they are a really useful way of using up leftover bits of salad from last night's dinner. The addition of za'atar and use of Persian lavash bread (now available in most mainstream supermarkets) gives the wraps an irresistible Middle Eastern twist.

1. Place the eggs in a small saucepan and top with kettle-hot water (if you've already made your morning tea or coffee the kettle is likely already full of just-boiled water). Place over a medium heat for 6 minutes before draining the eggs and peeling off the shells. I do this under cold running water for speed and ease.

2. Warm the lavash bread, either in the microwave for 20 seconds or in a dry frying pan (you can skip this step if you're short on time). Top the bread with the yoghurt, then slice the egg into quarters and place in the centre of the bread along with the cucumber, tomato, onion and za'atar. Season with a little salt, then roll into a tight wrap, slice in half and eat right away (or wrap in baking paper or foil if you are eating on the move).

 Time Saving Hack
If you are boiling the eggs in the morning, take them out of the fridge the night before so that they are room temperature when you start cooking them. You can also hard-boil your eggs the night before and have them ready for use in the morning, as well as prepping your cucumber, tomato and onion and keeping in a Tupperware container in the fridge.

Berry + Chia Seed Breakfast

Diversity points: 6 / Fibre: 16g

2 x 400g (14oz) tins coconut milk

400g (14oz) frozen mixed summer berries

4 tbsp jumbo oats

2 tbsp flaxseeds or linseeds

Seeds of 2 fat cardamom pods

2 tbsp maple syrup (optional)

100g (3½oz/¾ cup) chia seeds

Kefir yoghurt or other live yoghurt, to serve (optional)

+ Bonus Diversity Points
Serve topped with mixed nuts and seeds or extra berries.

One of the most popular recipes from my previous book, *The Kitchen Prescription*, was a mango and chia seed breakfast pudding. So here is another vibrant, yet inexpensive, chia-based breakfast recipe. It is surprisingly filling, probably because it is packed to the very brim with gut-loving fibre. I always advise eating chia seeds with water to get the maximum benefit, so have a large glass of water with this delight.

1. Add the coconut milk, frozen berries, oats, flaxseeds and cardamom seeds to a blender and blitz to a smooth purée. Frozen berries can sometimes be quite tart, so taste the mixture and add the maple syrup if you think it needs a touch of sweetness.

2. Pour the blended fruit mixture into a large bowl, add the chia seeds and stir everything well to combine. Refrigerate for a few hours, or overnight.

3. Serve with some kefir or live yoghurt, if you like.

Time Saving Hack
Use frozen mixed berries rather than trying to buy 3 or 4 different types of fresh berry: this will save you time and money. You can use mixed frozen tropical fruit, or any other combination that you like.

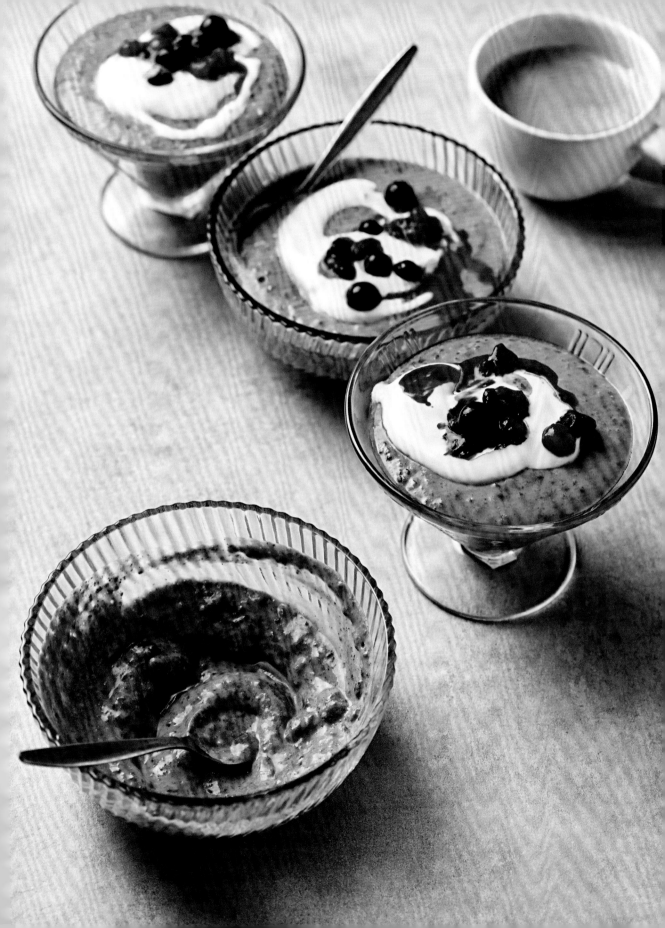

Avocado + Smoked Salmon Breakfast Salad

Diversity points: 5 / Fibre: 4.3g

Salad for breakfast, anyone? Smoked salmon and avocado is a classic breakfast combination which thankfully requires no cooking! This is a great way to use up any leftover salad leaves that are starting to wilt, especially when served with toasted slices of seedy bread. Adapt the recipe to whichever salad ingredients and herbs are sitting in the back of your fridge.

4 handfuls of baby spinach leaves

4 handfuls of watercress leaves

2 large ripe avocados

150g (5oz) smoked salmon

120g (4oz) feta cheese

12 toasted walnuts

2 tbsp olive oil

Juice of ½ lemon

Handful of soft herbs, such as mint, parsley, basil or dill, chopped (optional)

Chilli flakes (optional)

1. Divide the spinach and watercress leaves between four plates. Halve and stone the avocados, then use a spoon to scoop the flesh out over the spinach and watercress.

2. Roughly tear the smoked salmon and strew around the avocado and salad leaves.

3. Crumble over the feta cheese and walnuts and drizzle over the olive oil. Squeeze over a touch of lemon juice and season with herbs of your choice and chilli flakes (if using). No extra salt is required as the salmon and feta are already salty enough.

+ Bonus Diversity Points
Serve topped with mixed toasted seeds or add sliced cucumber and tomato. For extra protein, you can serve with eggs.

Time Saving Hack
You can prepare the salad the night before (without the feta) and have it waiting for you in a plastic container in the fridge. Just dress with olive oil and lemon juice and add the feta in the morning.

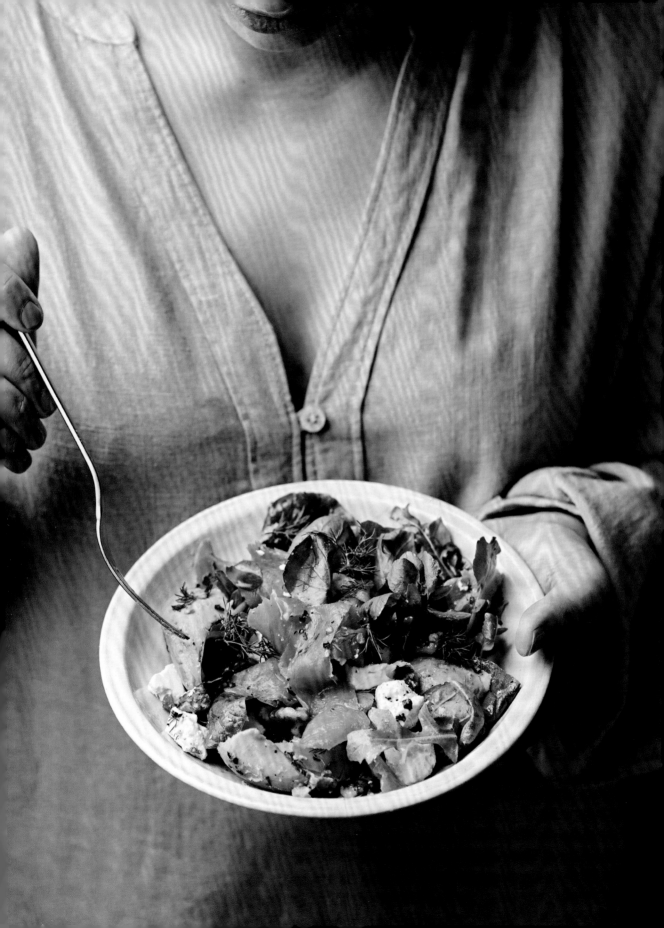

Instant Creamy Spinach + Chickpeas

Diversity points: 5 / Fibre: 12g

1 x 400g (14oz) tin chickpeas
100g (3½oz) frozen chopped spinach
2 tbsp extra-virgin olive oil, plus extra to drizzle
Juice of ½ lemon
2 tbsp full fat live Greek yoghurt
1 tbsp tahini
Handful of toasted pine nuts (optional)
½ tsp dried mint or za'atar (optional)
Wholewheat pitta bread, toasted
Salt, to taste

+ Bonus Diversity Points
Add finely chopped tomatoes, parsley and pomegranate seeds if you like. You can also serve the dish with some lacto-fermented vegetables, like cucumbers and turnips.

Savoury, protein-rich breakfasts are much more likely to keep us feeling fuller for longer, plus they are a great alternative to all the sweet breakfast options that we end up eating most of the time. No pots or pans are required here – the microwave does all the good work for you.

1. Drain the chickpeas and rinse them under cold running water. Tip them into a microwave-safe bowl, add the frozen chopped spinach and season with salt. Cover the bowl with a lid and microwave on high power for 3½ minutes.

2. Remove the chickpeas and spinach from the microwave and carefully take off the lid; it will be quite steamy, so take care. Add the olive oil, lemon juice, yoghurt and tahini and give the whole mixture a really good mix to combine.

3. Pour the chickpeas into a serving bowl and drizzle with a little more olive oil and, if you have them, the toasted pine nuts and dried mint. Serve with toasted pitta bread.

Time Saving Hack
You can have the chickpeas and spinach ready in your microwave-safe bowl the night before, so that you just have to pop them into the microwave for breakfast. You can even mix the lemon juice, yoghurt and tahini the night before and have it ready to pour on to the chickpeas the next morning.

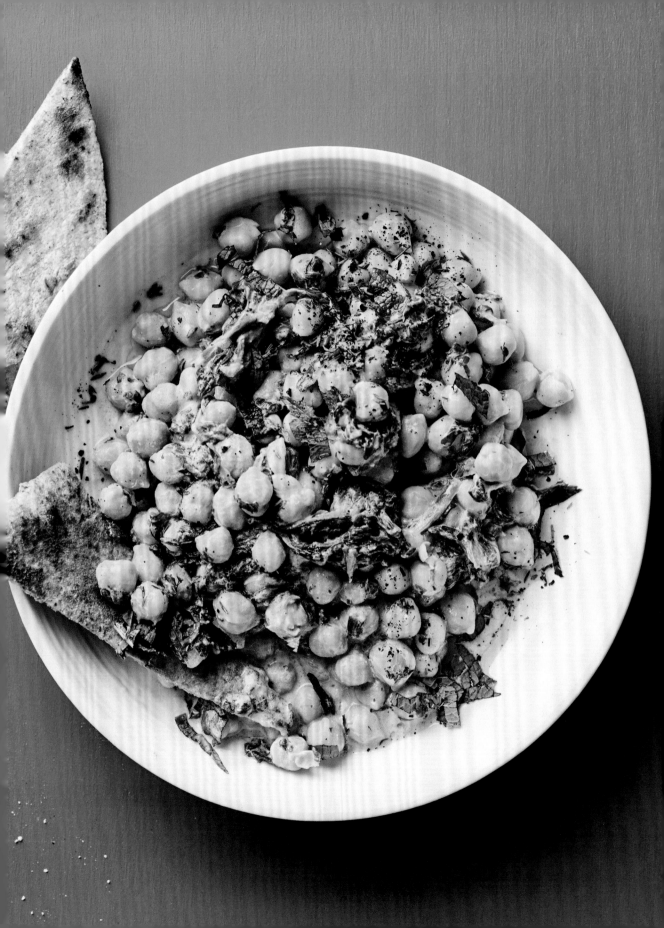

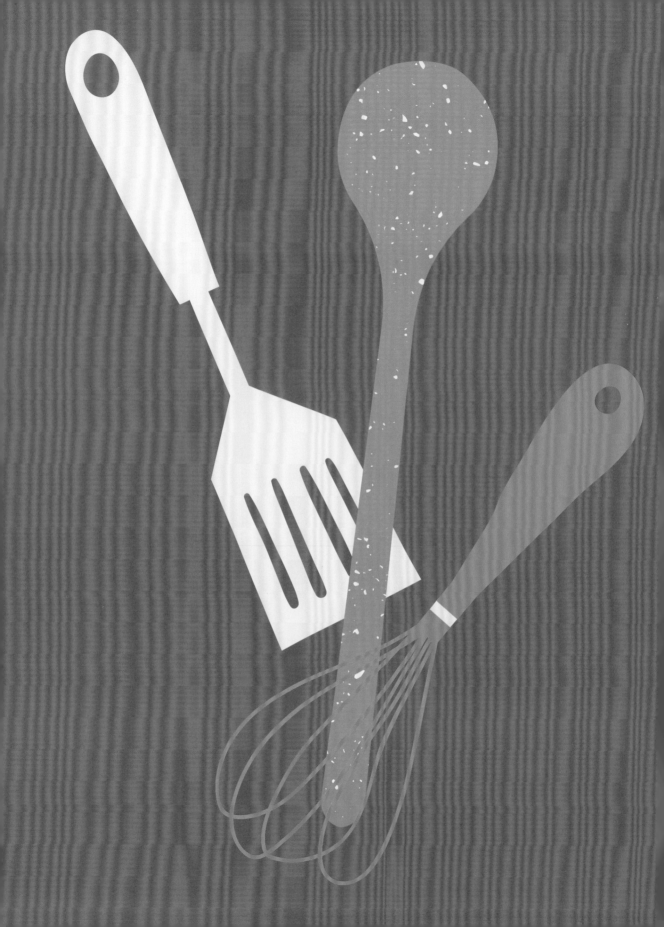

Easy Speedy Brunch

chapter two

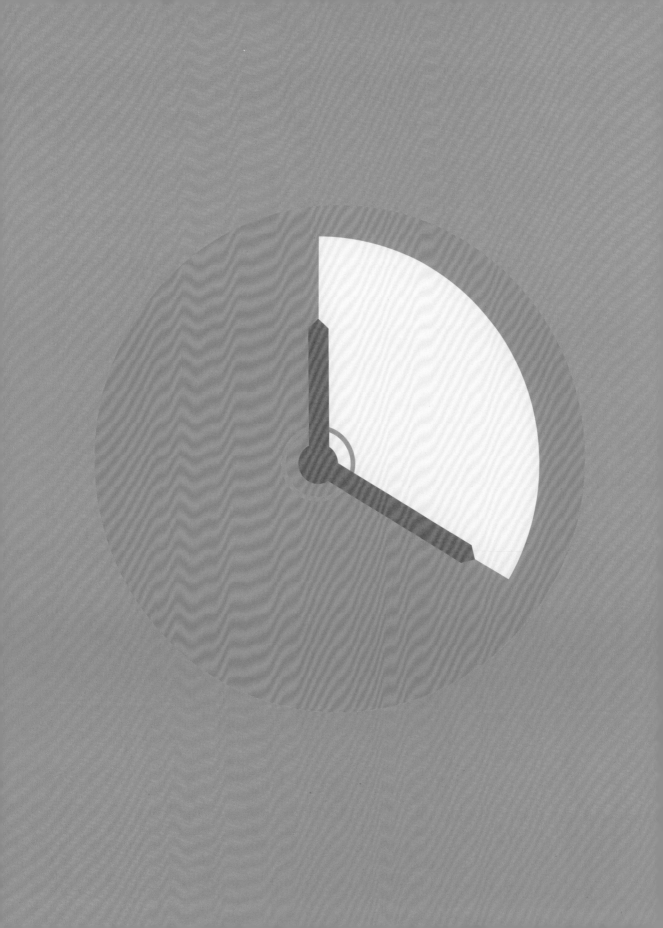

Brunch is one of those meals that sits in meal purgatory . . . is it a real meal, or just something made up by restaurants as an excuse to serve prosecco at 11 a.m.? For me, if breakfast is a mealtime, brunch is more of a culture; an opportunity to load up on gut-healthy ingredients in a relaxed, social setting; a way to put life's constant stress to one side for a couple of hours and enjoy great food with even greater company.

Life's trials and tribulations impact the delicate gut–brain relationship and can wreak havoc with the digestive system. Stress can worsen bloating, abdominal pain and reflux, lead to diarrhoea or constipation, and even exacerbate inflammation. So, any mealtime that can alleviate stress and lead to relaxation is well worth making time for. Mere mention of the word 'brunch' conjures up images of mindful, considered eating, surrounded by friends, family and loved ones . . . bliss.

Alongside this, brunch recipes lend themselves well to increasing our consumption of a diverse range of whole-food plant-based ingredients. Key elements of most brunches include fruit, salad, greenery; on reflection, it's probably harder to buy a pre-made, ultra-processed brunch off the supermarket shelf than to cook one from scratch yourself.

Eggs are also an essential component of the brunch table; egg recipes lend themselves well to being packed with vegetables, herbs and spices, and you'll always end up feeling comfortably full at the end of the meal. Spreadable toppings, seedy crackers and toast and beany dips are also endlessly versatile and a gut-healthy, non-labour-intensive way of making sure you maintain your position as the most popular brunch host among your friends.

Brunch benefits from simplicity. An uncluttered, uncomplicated brunch table is far more suited to the relaxed brunch ethos than an overengineered collection of napkins and six differently sized forks for each person. My brunch tables at home are proudly served on whatever clean plates and cutlery I can find, and you'll often find at least one person drinking from my son's plastic Minions cup. With brunch, presentation is far less important than substance.

For all these reasons, I thought that a chapter full of express brunch recipes might be useful to those of you seeking inspiration for your next weekend gathering. I've tried to balance a bit of indulgence with easy preparation and a hefty dose of gut-friendly nutrition. And as a bonus, these recipes can all be used make wonderful savoury breakfasts or light lunches in their own right, so don't worry if you aren't really a brunch person. Start experimenting and see what works best for you!

Miso Garlic Beans on Toast

Diversity points: 3 / Fibre: 16g (if serving 2)

1 x 400g (14oz) tin black-eyed peas

1 x 400g (14oz) tin white beans/cannellini beans

2 generous tbsp olive oil

2 tsp garlic paste from a jar (or 2 large garlic cloves, thinly sliced)

1 tsp tomato purée (optional)

2 tsp white miso paste

250ml (9fl oz/1 cup) kettle-hot water

Juice of ½ lemon

Handful of chives, finely chopped

1 heaped tsp chiu chow chilli oil

TO SERVE

4 slices of seedy sourdough bread

Kimchi (optional)

+ Bonus Diversity Points

Use different combinations of tinned beans/lentils each time you make this recipe to optimise diversity.

A versatile, umami bomb of a recipe that uses any tinned beans in your pantry: cannellini beans, chickpeas and kidney beans all work exceptionally well when given the garlic and miso treatment. Serve alongside toasted seedy bread and extra probiotic kimchi if you wish.

1. Put the kettle on to boil. Drain the black-eyed peas and cannellini beans in a colander and rinse through quickly with cold water.

2. Place a wide frying pan over a medium heat. Add the olive oil and garlic to the pan and sauté the garlic for just a minute until it starts to turn golden brown and release its aroma. Add the tomato purée and miso paste, followed a minute later by the black-eyed peas and cannellini beans. Stir everything well to combine, then add the kettle-hot water and lemon juice. Simmer for another 3–5 minutes to reduce the mixture down slightly. You can reduce the beans down completely if you wish; I prefer to keep them a bit looser and spoonable.

3. To serve, sprinkle over the chives and the chilli oil. Enjoy with seedy toasted bread and a spoonful of kimchi (if using).

Time Saving Hack

Use pre-minced garlic from a jar instead of peeling and mincing cloves from scratch yourself. You can also buy frozen minced garlic, which works really well. If you are feeling super organised, you can even drain and wash the beans the night before and keep them ready for use in a Tupperware container in the fridge. A wide, shallow pan rather than a deep saucepan will speed up cooking time significantly as water evaporates out faster from a wide pan.

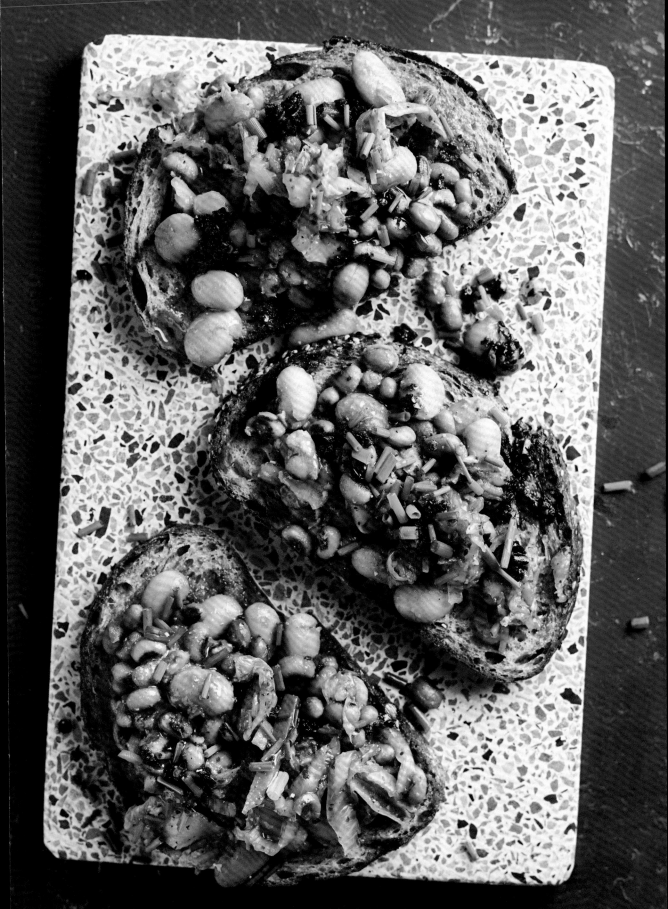

Lemon + Herb Chickpeas + Quinoa

Diversity points: 8 / Fibre: 18g

2 x 400g (14oz) tins chickpeas

250g (9oz) pre-cooked quinoa (from a pouch)

4 tbsp extra-virgin olive oil, plus extra to drizzle

2 large, ripe tomatoes, diced

Large handful of parsley, finely chopped

Large handful of coriander, finely chopped

Juice of 1 lemon

1 tsp cumin seeds

1 tsp red chilli flakes

500g (1lb 2oz) full-fat live Greek yoghurt

4 heaped tbsp tahini

1 tsp garlic paste from a jar

4 tbsp pomegranate seeds

Salt to taste

+ Bonus Diversity Points

Add grated cauliflower, broccoli, diced onions, cucumbers and radishes for added plant diversity. Or why not top with extra toasted pine nuts and seeds?

Brunch, but with Middle Eastern vibes. I often make this dish for friends and they are always impressed at how much energy I have put in to preparing this for them . . . little do they know how effortlessly simple this dish really is. Just ten minutes from kitchen to table, with a little help from the microwave.

1. Drain and rinse the chickpeas in a colander and place them in a large microwave-safe bowl together with the cooked quinoa. Drizzle over a splash of water, cover the microwave-safe bowl with a lid and microwave for 2 ½ minutes till piping hot.

2. Remove the chickpeas and quinoa from the microwave and drizzle over the olive oil and add the tomatoes and herbs. Season the chickpea and quinoa mixture with the lemon juice, cumin seeds and red chilli flakes as well as a generous pinch of salt. Stir everything really well to combine.

3. To complete the dish, mix the yoghurt, tahini and garlic together in a large bowl with a pinch of salt. To serve, spoon large dollops of the yoghurt over the quinoa and scatter over pomegranate seeds, any leftover herbs and a further drizzle of olive oil.

Time Saving Hack
I use pre-cooked quinoa straight from a pouch to save time in this recipe, though you can use any other pre-made grain from a pouch, or grains that you have prepared in advance and refrigerated. Leftover wild rice, pearl barley or bulgur wheat would also serve as a great substitute for quinoa. Removing seeds from a pomegranate can be fiddly and messy, so I use pre-prepared packets of pomegranate seeds.

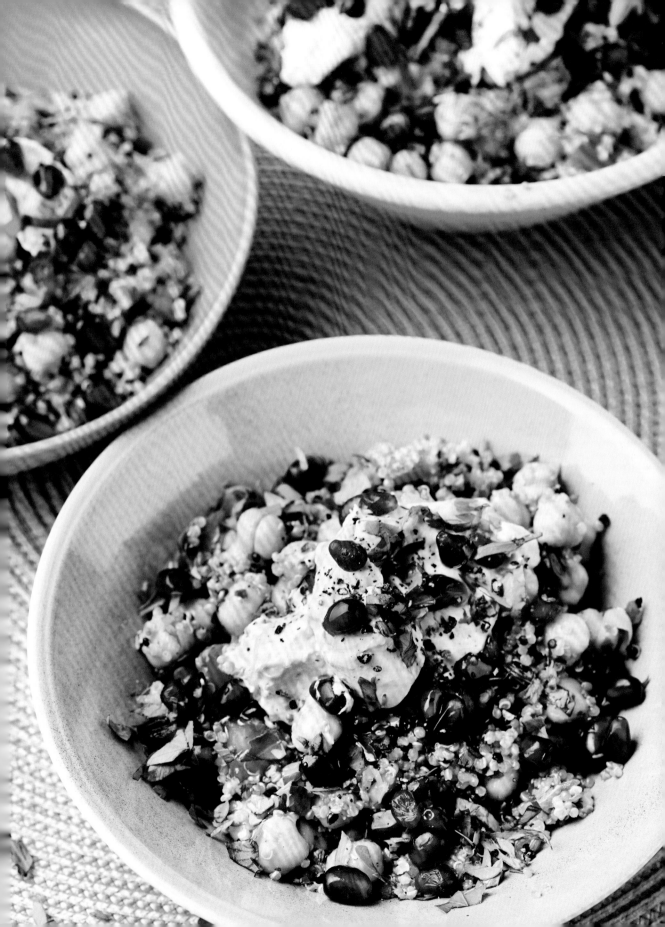

Spiced Tofu Spinach Scramble

Diversity points: 4 / Fibre: 6.8g

300g (10oz) spinach leaves
4 generous tbsp vegetable oil
1 large red onion, diced
2 tsp cumin seeds
2 tsp ground turmeric
2 tsp red chilli flakes
2 x 400g (14oz) blocks of firm tofu
2 tbsp nutritional yeast
1 tsp black salt

+ Bonus Diversity Points

Add sautéed mushrooms or red and yellow peppers and extra cherry tomatoes.

I had to feature a vegan alternative to eggs on account of how many newly converted vegans dearly miss eating them. The trick is to use black salt and nutritional yeast to impart that slightly sulphurous 'eggy' tang, and to be generous with the spicing as tofu really does need heaps of seasoning to make it taste good.

1. Take a large non-stick frying pan and place it over a high heat. Add the spinach and a splash of water and cook until the leaves have just wilted; this will only take a minute or so. Tip the spinach out on to a plate and set aside.

2. Return the pan to the heat and drizzle in the oil. Add the diced onion and sauté for just 2 minutes to soften, then add the cumin seeds, turmeric and chilli flakes. Now add the tofu, broken down by hand into small chunks. Stir everything well so that the tofu evenly takes on the yellow hue of the turmeric. Season the tofu with nutritional yeast and black salt before returning the wilted spinach to the pan. Stir through, then serve immediately.

 Time Saving Hack
If you are in a rush, you can omit the onion from this recipe. Simply add the spices to the oil, followed by the tofu.

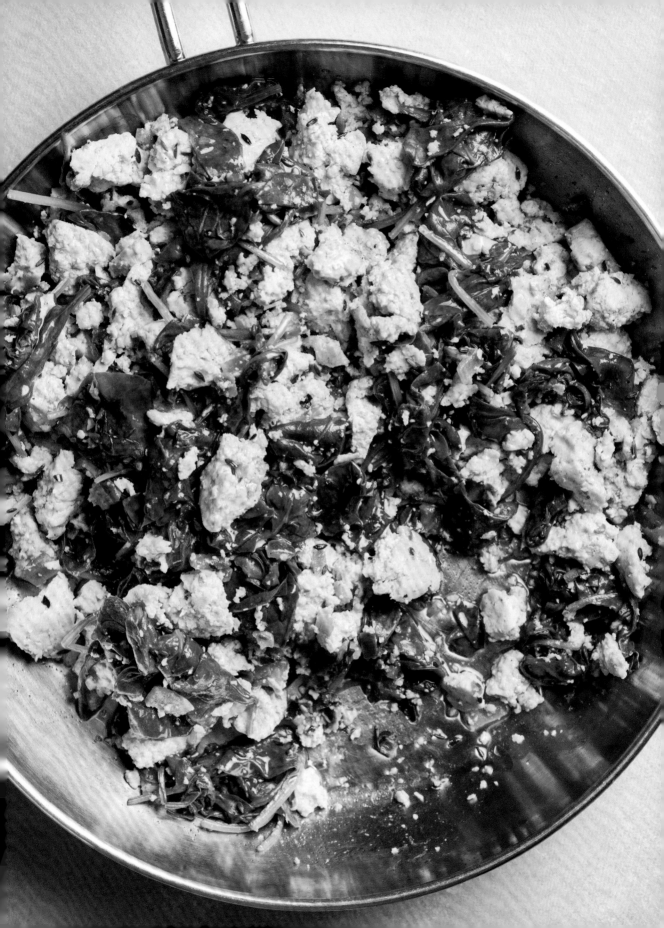

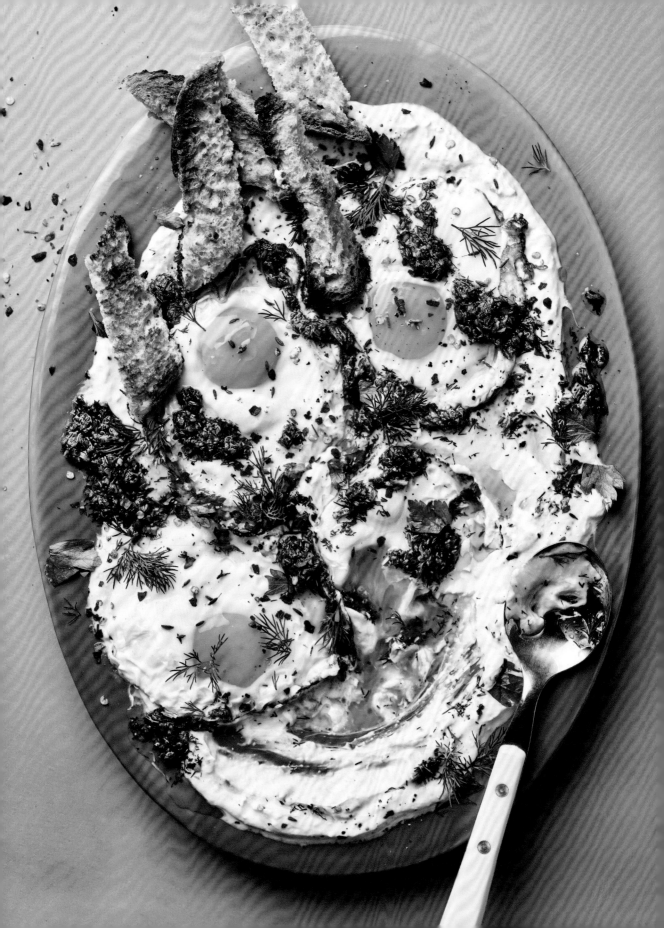

Eggs + Garlicky Yoghurt with Zingy Green Sauce

Diversity points: 3 / Fibre: 5.2g

2 tbsp vegetable oil

4 large free-range eggs

400g (14oz) full-fat live Greek yoghurt

4 tsp garlic paste from a jar

4 slices of sourdough or bread of your choice

25g (1oz) dill

25g (1oz) parsley

4 tbsp extra-virgin oil

Juice of ½ lemon

½ tsp red chilli flakes

Salt, to taste

+ Bonus Diversity Points

Boost plant diversity by adding spring onions and spinach leaves to your herby sauce. You can also spoon tinned green lentils over the yoghurt before topping with your eggs.

This recipe is similar to Turkish eggs, but substitutes the chilli butter with a zippy, lip-smacking salsa verde-style sauce. Crisp toasted chunks of bread are great for dipping into the runny yolk and zingy sauce. Green tea would be a perfect side.

1. Place a small pan over a medium heat and add the vegetable oil. When the oil is hot but not smoking, carefully crack in the eggs and fry them until the whites are cooked but the yolks remain runny. Set aside.

2. Mix the yoghurt and half the garlic together and season with salt to taste. Spread this yoghurt mixture out on to a shallow platter, then carefully place the eggs over the yoghurt, taking care not to break the yolks. Season the eggs with salt and place the bread into the toaster.

3. To make the herby sauce, add the herbs and remaining garlic to a food processor and blitz until the herbs are finely chopped. Add the olive oil, lemon juice and chilli flakes to the blitzed herbs and season with salt to taste. Mix well and spoon the herby sauce over the eggs.

4. Serve the dish with toast, cut into chunky soldiers for dipping.

 Time Saving Hack
Make double the quantity of the herby sauce and store the leftover sauce in the fridge. Use it to dress roasted peppers or to spoon over burrata, or to make a pasta salad tossed through with extra nuts and seeds.

Fruity Brunch Couscous

Diversity points: 4 / Fibre: 4.9g

100g (3½oz/½ cup) dried couscous

150g (4oz) strawberries, hulled and sliced or quartered

2 tbsp pistachios, roughly chopped

2 handfuls of parsley, roughly chopped

1 tbsp maple syrup

2 tbsp extra-virgin olive oil

1 tbsp balsamic vinegar or pomegranate molasses

2 tbsp pumpkin seeds

75g (2¾oz) goats' cheese, crumbled

Salt, to taste

+ Bonus Diversity Points
Adding a handful of dark leafy greens (rocket, watercress or spinach) would work well.

Couscous for brunch, I hear you ask? Yes, yes, yes. It really does work! This fruity, nutty combination is perfect with salty, crumbled goats' cheese. You can use blueberries, ripe peaches and raspberries or even blackberries instead of strawberries if you like.

1. Tip the dried couscous into a large bowl and cover with boiling water from the kettle until it comes to just a centimetre above the couscous. Cover the bowl with a plate and set aside for 5–10 minutes while you prepare the strawberries, pistachios and parsley.

2. Fluff up the couscous with a fork and add the maple syrup, extra-virgin olive oil and season with salt to taste. Stir the couscous really well before tossing in the strawberries, pistachios and parsley.

3. To complete the dish, drizzle over the balsamic vinegar and scatter over the pumpkin seeds and crumbled goats' cheese.

 Time Saving Hack
Use any pre-cooked grain from your fridge instead of making fresh couscous or use pouches of pre-cooked grains – quinoa, pearl barley and spelt would all work very well.

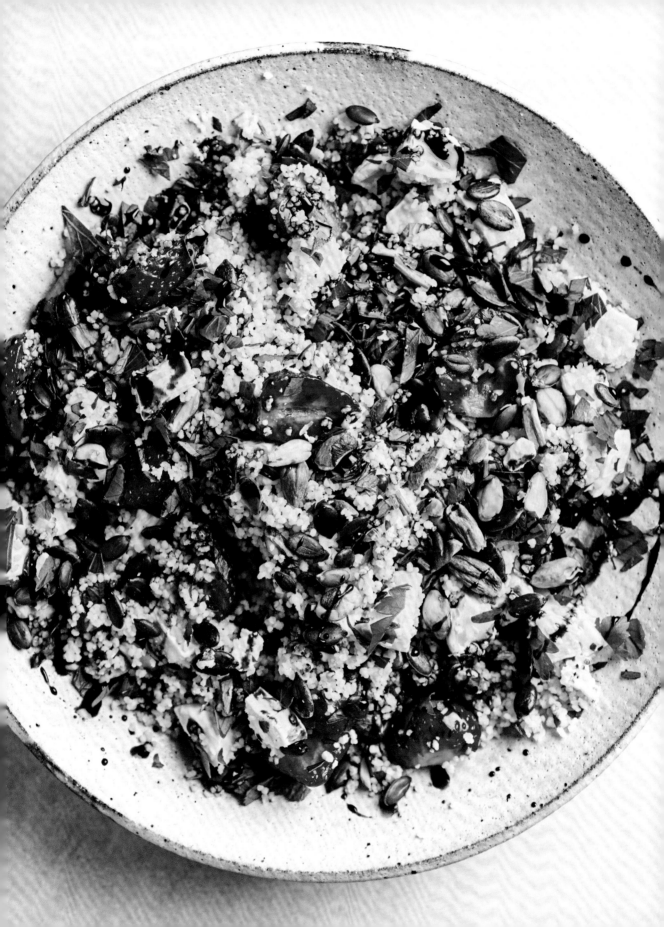

Easy 'Peasy' Pancakes

Diversity points: 3 / Fibre: 3.3g

125g (4oz) cottage cheese

200g (7oz) frozen petits pois, defrosted

Handful of spinach leaves

1 tsp cumin seeds

½ tsp garam masala

½ tsp red chilli powder or flakes

120ml (4fl oz/½ cup) whole milk

2 eggs

4 tbsp cornflour

½ tsp bicarbonate of soda

½ tsp baking powder

Vegetable oil

Salt, to taste

TO SERVE (OPTIONAL)

2–3 tbsp full-fat live Greek yoghurt

Lime pickle

+ Bonus Diversity Points

Boost plant diversity by adding herbs like parsley and coriander to the pancake batter.

Vibrant green pancakes pair really well with some extra chilli pickle and cooling yoghurt. Adding cottage cheese and peas serves to boost the protein content of these pancakes, and this may well help keep you fuller for longer.

1. Add the cottage cheese, petits pois, spinach, cumin seeds, garam masala, red chilli powder and milk to a blender and blitz to a smooth purée.

2. Now add the eggs, cornflour, bicarbonate of soda and baking powder to the blender along with salt to taste and blend once again until all the ingredients are incorporated.

3. Place a good non-stick pan over a medium heat and brush it with a teaspoon of vegetable oil. Gently pour enough pancake batter gently into the pan to form a pancake about 10–12cm (4–5in) in diameter and 5mm (¼in) thick. I usually cook two to three in the pan at the same time.

4. When bubbles start appearing on the surface of the pancakes (after about 2 minutes) and they look just set, carefully flip them over with a palette knife. The batter is sticky so don't rush. Cook for a further minute or so until the pancakes are cooked through, then keep aside on a plate. The mixture should make around 8 or so pancakes. Serve the pancakes with some cooling yoghurt and lime pickle if you wish.

Time Saving Hack

There's no need to pour the batter from the blender into a pouring jug before cooking the pancakes – just drop the batter straight from the blender into the pan.

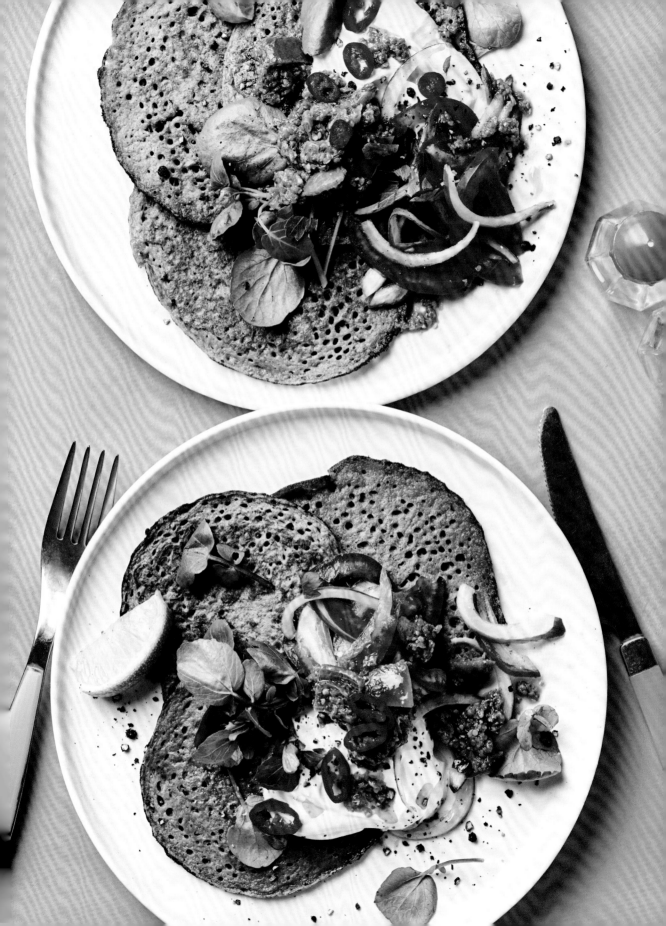

Scrambled Eggs + Greens

Diversity points: 4 / Fibre: 3.2g

200g (7oz) Tenderstem broccoli, chopped into 2cm (¾in) lengths

75g (2¾oz) curly kale from a pack, cut and washed

75g (2¾oz) frozen peas

1 tbsp vegetable oil

6 eggs

2 tsp sesame oil

1 tbsp soy sauce or kecap manis

1 tsp chilli oil, or to taste

1 tsp black sesame seeds

Salt, to taste

+ Bonus Diversity Points
Add extra greens, like runner beans, pak choi, edamame beans, okra and spring onions in addition to the vegetables used here.

How do you like your eggs in the morning? I like mine scrambled with greens! Soft, sesame-spiked eggs really are the perfect vessel for vibrant crisp green vegetables. You can, of course, use any green vegetables at your disposal; from green beans to mangetout or even pak choi, there's a whole world of greens out there.

1. Put the broccoli, kale and peas into a large frying pan and splash over a few tablespoons of water. Place the lid on the pan and steam the vegetables for about 3 minutes until they have just cooked through but remain crisp and still a vibrant green.

2. Place another medium non-stick frying pan over a medium heat with a tablespoon of vegetable oil. Crack the eggs into a bowl, add the sesame oil and season with salt to taste, then whisk together to combine. Pour the eggs into the frying pan and cook through to a very soft, scrambled consistency, about 2 minutes.

3. Tip the eggs out of the pan and into a wide-mouthed bowl. Arrange the steamed greens on top and drizzle over the soy sauce or kecap manis, chilli oil and sesame seeds. Serve immediately – leftover rice, cooked and cooled the day before, would make a fantastic accompaniment.

 Time Saving Hack
Have your green vegetables cut and ready for use the night before and keep in a Tupperware container. You can even use leftover cooked greens from dinner the night before in this recipe.

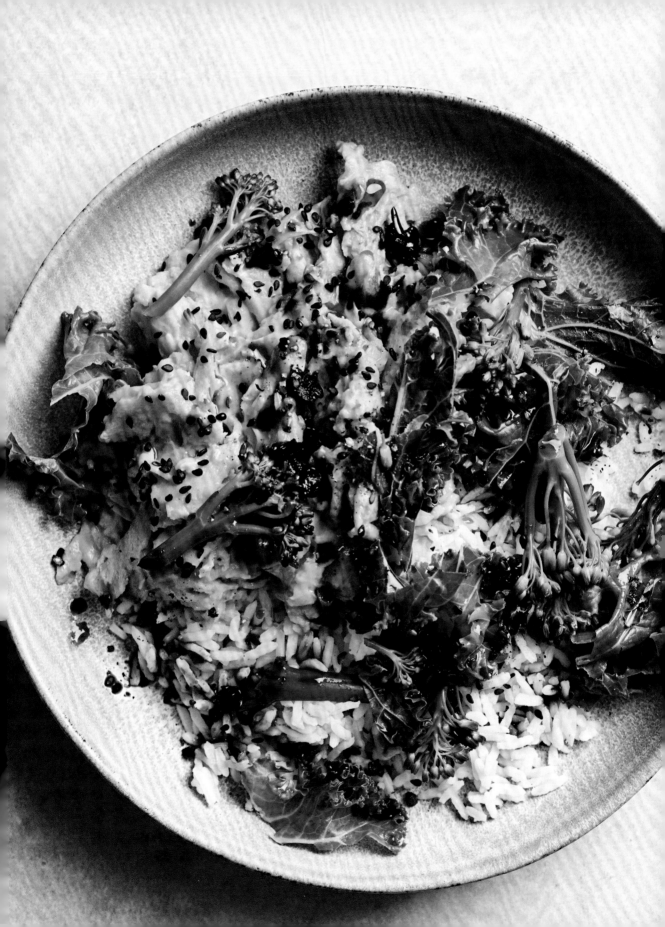

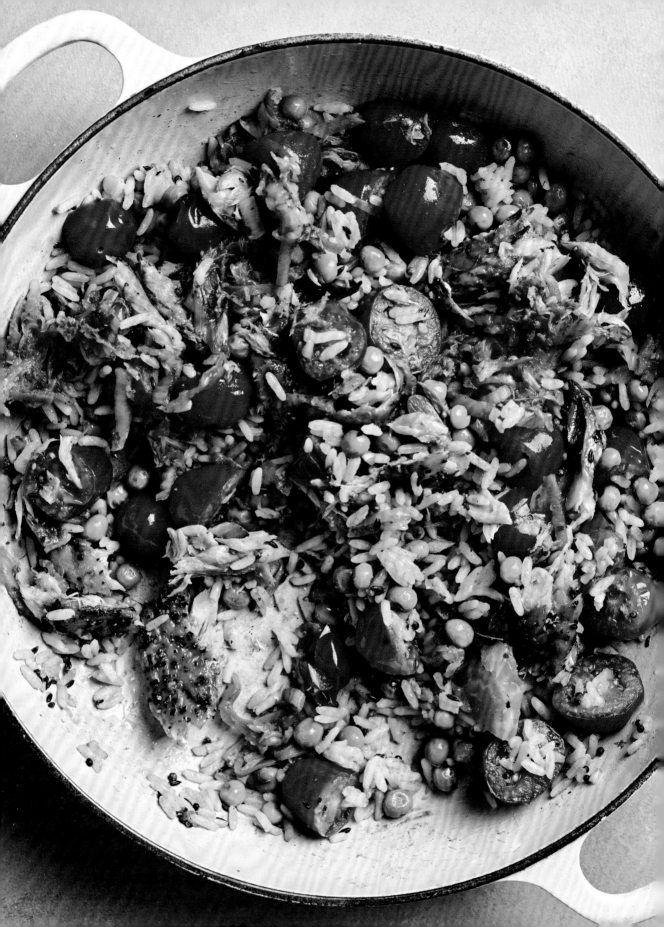

Kimchi + Mackerel Kedgeree

SERVES 2
(WITH LEFTOVERS)

Diversity points: 4 / Fibre: 4.1g

2 generous tbsp olive oil

1 tsp cumin seeds

½ tsp ground turmeric

1 tsp mustard seeds

½ tsp red chilli powder

180g (6oz) frozen petits pois

250g (9oz) pouch pre-cooked basmati rice

200g (7oz) cherry tomatoes, halved

2 fillets of smoked mackerel (200g/7oz)

100g (3½oz) kimchi and its juice, plus extra to serve alongside

Salt, to taste

+ Bonus Diversity Points

Add diced green spring onions to the hot oil before adding spices for a few extra diversity points. Garlic and ginger also make a worthy addition. Serve with boiled eggs for increased protein content.

Kedgeree, of sorts, but with an extra gut-loving probiotic kimchi boost. Mackerel is such an under-utilised oily fish. I love its full-bodied flavour and the fact that it is rich in beneficial anti-inflammatory omega oils. This is particularly special for cold wintery brunches – just double up the quantities to serve four.

1. Place a large frying pan or wok over a medium heat and add the olive oil. When the oil is hot, but not smoking, add the cumin seeds, turmeric, mustard seeds and red chilli powder, followed quickly by the petits pois. Stir everything well to combine and cook for a minute or two, by which time the peas will have defrosted.

2. Now add the rice from the packet and a few splashes of water. Cook for a further 2 minutes before tossing in the tomatoes, then season with salt and once again stir everything well.

3. To complete the dish, remove the skin from the mackerel and flake it on to the rice. Top with the kimchi and its juice and serve immediately.

 Time Saving Hack
Pre-cooked rice in a pouch is a saviour here, as are garden peas which I use straight from the freezer. To save time, you can defrost the peas in the microwave before adding them to the dish.

Garlicky Fava Bean Dip with Crudités

Diversity points: 5 (for the dip, 6 more for crudites) / Fibre: 9.2g

2 x 400g (14oz) tins fava beans

2–3 garlic cloves

3 tbsp tahini

1 tsp chilli flakes

1 tsp cumin seeds

3 tbsp extra-virgin olive oil, plus extra for drizzling

Juice of 1 lemon

Handful of parsley

1 spring onion, roughly chopped

TO SERVE

Toasted sourdough bread

Seedy wholewheat crackers

Handful of pink radishes

Handful of baby cucumbers, sliced lengthways

Handful of carrot batons

Handful of celery sticks

Handful of radicchio or endive leaves

Handful of mangetout

+ Bonus Diversity Points

Use another bean instead of fava beans to the dip – cannellini or butter beans would also work well. Use as many different vegetables in your crudités as possible, maybe sprinkling them with extra sumac and za'atar for interest.

Dare I say this is the new hummus! Nowadays tinned fava beans are stocked in nearly all supermarkets in the World Food sections. They are the meatiest of all beans, creamy and fibre-dense in equal measure, although any tinned bean would work perfectly here.

1. Bring a kettle of water to the boil. Drain the fava beans and rinse them through with some kettle-hot water. Place the warmed beans in a food processor with a few tablespoons of kettle-hot water, the garlic cloves, tahini, chilli flakes, cumin seeds, olive oil and lemon juice. Blitz to a rough purée – I prefer to keep it a bit coarse. Now add the parsley and spring onion and give the mixture another quick blitz to break down the parsley and spring onion.

2. Use a spatula to scrape all the dip from the food processor into a deep bowl. Drizzle over a little more olive, then serve with a selection of breads, crackers and vegetables. I've made some suggestions but use whichever vegetables you really like to go alongside the dip.

Time Saving Hack
The food processor does all the work here so that you don't have to. By running boiling water over the beans before blitzing them, you get a smoother result overall.

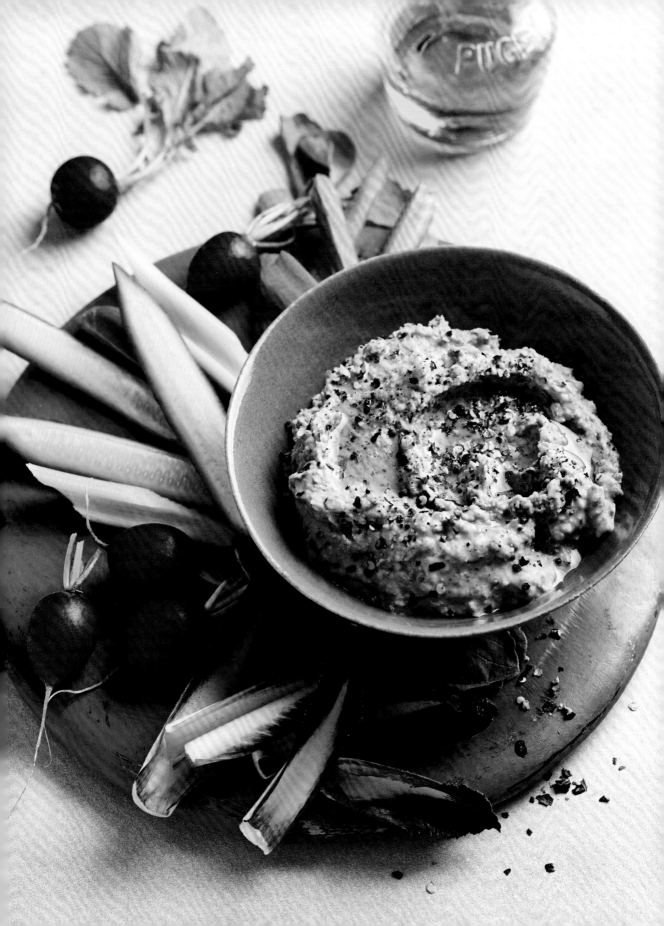

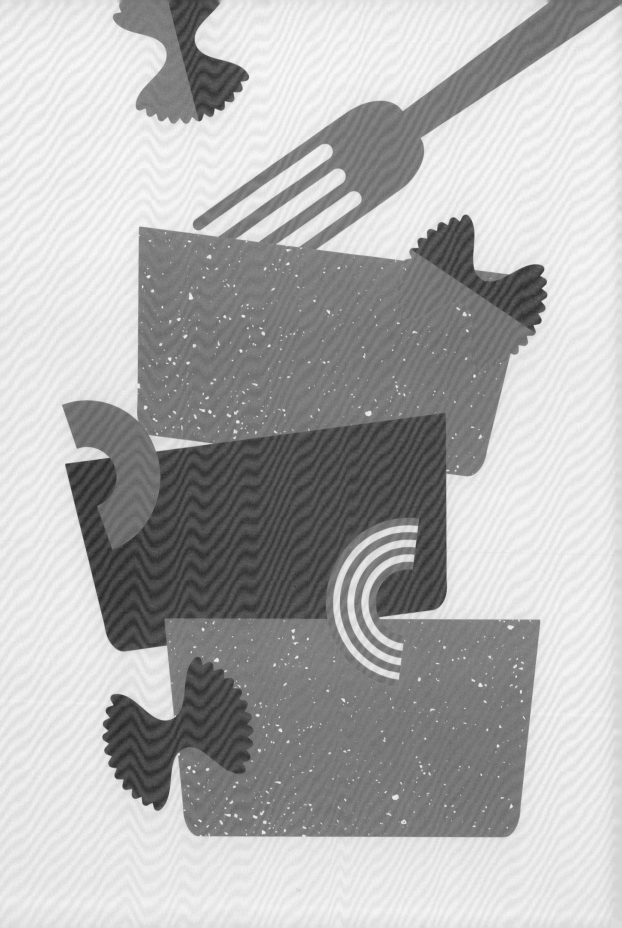

Lunch Express

chapter three

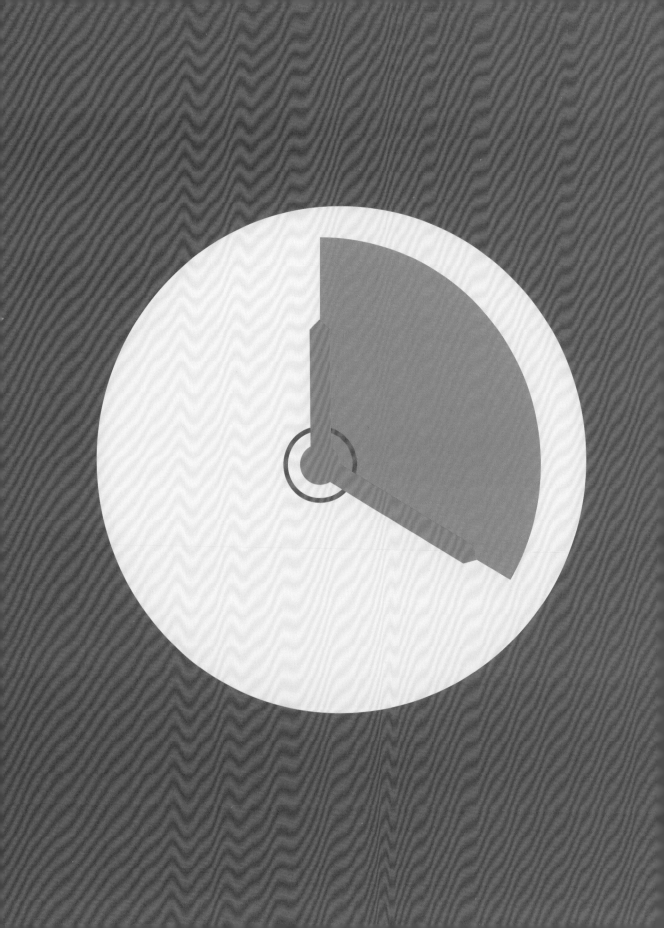

The late, great Orson Welles once said, 'Ask not what you can do for your country. Ask what's for lunch.' Now, Orson may well have been a man whose lunch was mostly prepared by someone else, but for the rest of us, do we ask ourselves what lunch is, or do we ask ourselves what lunch *should* be?

Some years ago, I found myself in a rut. Every lunchtime, I would buy the dullest meal deals from the local supermarket next to the NHS hospital I was working at as a junior doctor. At first, I tried to force myself to go for the 'healthier' options on the lunch shelves, but I slowly found myself reaching more and more for the ultra-processed food items (though at the time I didn't realise quite how processed these options were). As a result, I was spending not insignificant amounts of money each week on flavourless sandwiches and sugary drinks, only to feel hungry again an hour later.

There were also days where I would skip lunch completely. Now, as any of you who have been forced to skip lunch due to a busy job will know, this is by far the easiest way to guarantee that your afternoon will be unenjoyable at best; even worse, it will almost certainly derail any productivity you enjoyed in the morning.

However, it was the influence of one particularly food obsessed colleague that made me look more closely at my relationship with lunch. At 10 in the morning, during the ward round when we were visiting patients, booking scans and carrying out blood tests, she would be whispering sweet nothings into my ear like, 'When do you think we'll be able to eat our lunch?' and 'I brought an incredible lunch in today!' or the timeless classic, 'Is anyone else starving?'

The curious thing was that her insistence on making time for lunch did not make her less productive; in fact the opposite was true.

When we set aside time to eat lunch, we were far more likely to do all our work and leave hospital on time than if we had worked through our lunch break. Yes, dear reader, the 'working lunch' is a myth: people are far more productive when their bellies are satisfied.

I have designed the recipes in this chapter to encourage everyone to make a commitment to a more enjoyable lunchtime. To make things easier, I've split this chapter into two sections. The first focuses on 'Grab + Go' portable lunch ideas, recipes designed to be batch-cooked or prepared ahead of time (in no more than 20 minutes), resulting in meals that are effortlessly portable and ideal for stuffing into a Tupperware and dropping into your bag in the mornings.

The second genre of lunch recipes are for preparing at lunchtime, in your home. The COVID-19 pandemic inexorably changed our working patterns, with many of us now working more flexibly. The downside is that we often blur the lines between home and the workplace, so these recipes have been designed to restrengthen our work–home balance, and to remind ourselves that eating at home has the potential to be a joyful uplifting experience, not just a slice of toast in between Zoom calls.

These recipes also try to incorporate some core foundations that I believe a good lunch is built on. Firstly, try – if you can – to have at least one fermented item a day at lunch. Sauerkraut, kimchi, lacto-fermented cucumbers or kombucha are all ideal candidates. Secondly, make sure you hydrate yourself as well as eating your meal. Finally, and although not food-related, try to squeeze in a short burst of physical activity to help get the blood recirculating, particularly if your work is more desk-based. And when the weather permits, see if you can eat lunch outdoors – your body will thank you for choosing alfresco dining over (sorry) aldesko dining.

Chicken, Cucumber + Kimchi Sandwiches

Grab + Go
Lunch

Diversity points: 3 / Fibre: 8.5g

200g (7oz) cooked chicken, diced

2 heaped tbsp organic mayo, plus a little extra

2 spring onions, thinly sliced

12cm (5in) piece of cucumber

4 slices of brown, seedy bread

125g (4oz) kimchi, roughly chopped

Salt, to taste

+ Bonus Diversity Points
Add grated carrot, rocket leaves and tomato slices to your sandwich.

A lovely way of incorporating probiotic kimchi into your lunchtime routine. I use brown, seedy bread here, but you can use sourdough, rye bread, wholewheat pitta bread or any other wholemeal wraps of your choice. The chicken can be substituted for chickpeas for a vegetarian alternative.

1. Combine the chicken with the mayonnaise, spring onions and a touch of salt.

2. Halve the cucumber lengthways and deseed it – I use a teaspoon to scoop out the watery centre – then slice it into thin half-moons.

3. Toast the slices of bread till light golden brown.

4. To assemble the sandwich, divide the chicken between two slices of bread and then top with kimchi followed by cucumbers. Spread a tiny bit of mayonnaise onto the other two slices of bread and use these as the lid of the sandwiches. Press down firmly before slicing each sandwich in half, wrapping tightly in clingfilm or foil and taking to work with you.

Time Saving Hack
Make the chicken sandwich filling the night before and keep it in the fridge ready to assemble your sandwiches the next day.

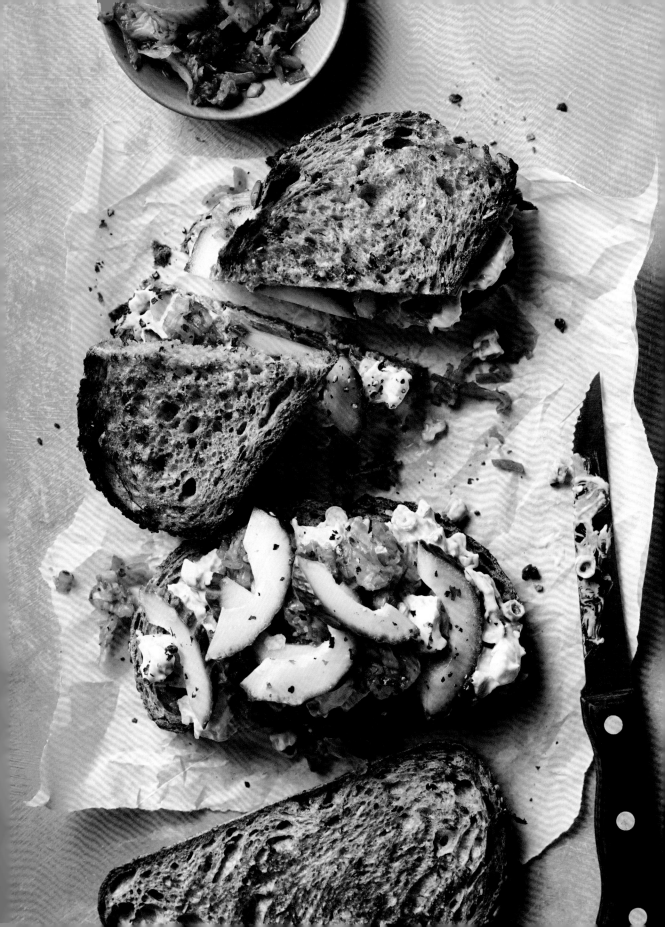

Pink Pasta

Diversity points: 4 / Fibre: 4.6g

200g (7oz) macaroni pasta

250g (9oz) cooked beetroot and the juice that comes inside the vacuum pack

200g (7oz) feta cheese

1 tbsp jalapeños from a jar

2 tbsp extra virgin olive oil

1 tbsp balsamic vinegar

1 tsp sumac (optional)

75g pistachio nut kernels, roughly chopped (optional)

Pomegranate seeds (optional)

Salt to taste

+ Bonus Diversity Points
Serve with leafy greens, chopped cucumbers and finely chopped parsley.

One of my favourite pasta salad recipes, on account not just of how utterly addictive it tastes, but also its retro fabulous pinky-mauve tinted colour. Beetroot is packed full of polyphenolic compounds and nitrates which help regulate blood flow and blood pressure. Cooking and cooling pasta helps develop resistant starch fibres in the pasta, which assists with slow release of energy, preparing you for the afternoon ahead.

1. Place a kettle on the boil. Pour the boiling hot water from the kettle into a saucepan and add the macaroni along with a heavy pinch of salt. Boil for 6-8 minutes as per packet instructions.

2. While the pasta is boiling, place the beetroot and its juice, feta, jalapeños, olive oil, vinegar and around half a cup of pasta water in a blender and blitz to a smooth purée.

3. When it has cooked through, drain the pasta and place it in large bowl. Pour over the beetroot sauce and mix well so that all the pasta is coated. Spoon the pasta into four Tupperware boxes and top with the sumac, the pistachio kernels and pomegranate seeds. Allow to cool before refrigerating.

Time Saving Hack
Use a small pasta like macaroni or orzo to reduce cooking time. Thankfully the pasta sauce is 'no cook' so it is super speedy to put together, just let your blender do all the work.

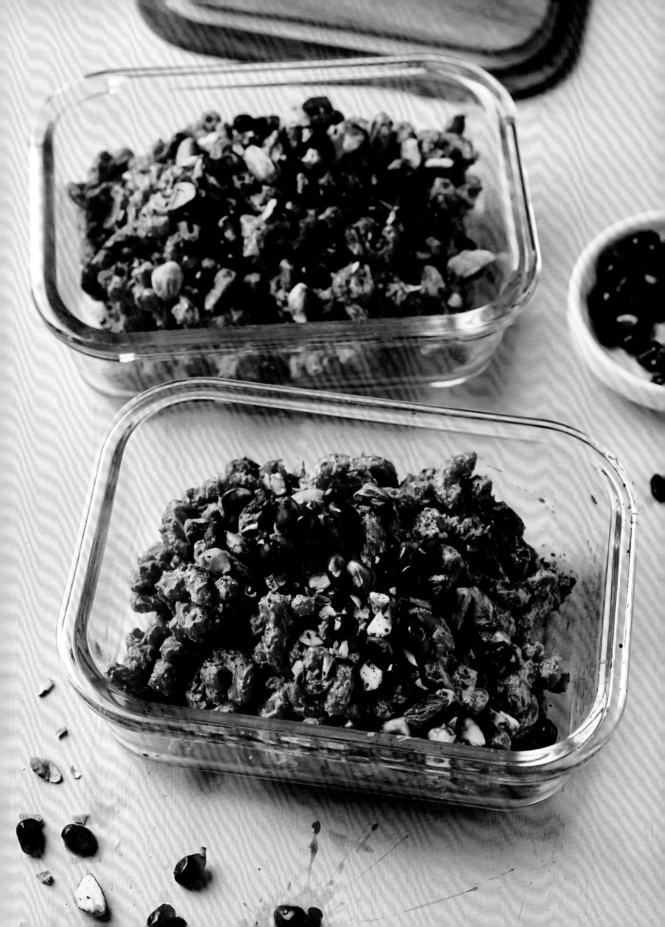

Peri Peri
Potato Salad

Grab + Go
Lunch

Diversity points: 7 / Fibre: 7.7g

1kg (2lb 4oz) pre-cooked baby new potatoes
150g (5oz) jarred peppers, roughly chopped
½ red onion, thinly sliced
1 x 198g (7oz) tin sweetcorn, drained (165g/5½oz drained weight)
2 heaped tsp peri peri rub (or 3 tbsp peri peri sauce)
1 tsp smoked paprika
3 tbsp full-fat live Greek yoghurt
Juice of 1 lime
2 tbsp olive oil
Handful of coriander, roughly chopped (optional)
Jalapeños from a jar (optional)
Salt, to taste

+ Bonus Diversity Points

Serve with a side of peas or some extra salad leaves of your choice. Look for a peri peri sauce that has no added E numbers or preservatives. If you can't find one, peri peri rubs are just spice mixes which don't have all the other additives, so are not classified as ultra-processed food items.

Here's a little tip for boosting fibre intake from your tatties: always keep the skin on and enjoy them cooked and then cooled; this helps develop the resistant starch that results in a slower release of energy. I like having these lip-smacking spicy potatoes with leftover roast chicken.

1. Cut the potatoes into quarters, keeping the skins on, and place in a large bowl. Add the chopped peppers and sliced red onion along with the sweetcorn, peri peri rub, paprika, yoghurt, lime juice and olive oil.

2. Season with salt to taste and mix everything really well to combine. Portion the potato salad into Tupperware containers and scatter over some chopped coriander and sliced jalapeños (if using). Refrigerate ready for use (it will keep for a good few days in the fridge).

Time Saving Hack

I often boil potatoes on a Sunday night, cool them and keep them refrigerated for use in various dishes in the week. It's a fantastic time-saving strategy, which you can replicate for various grains as well.

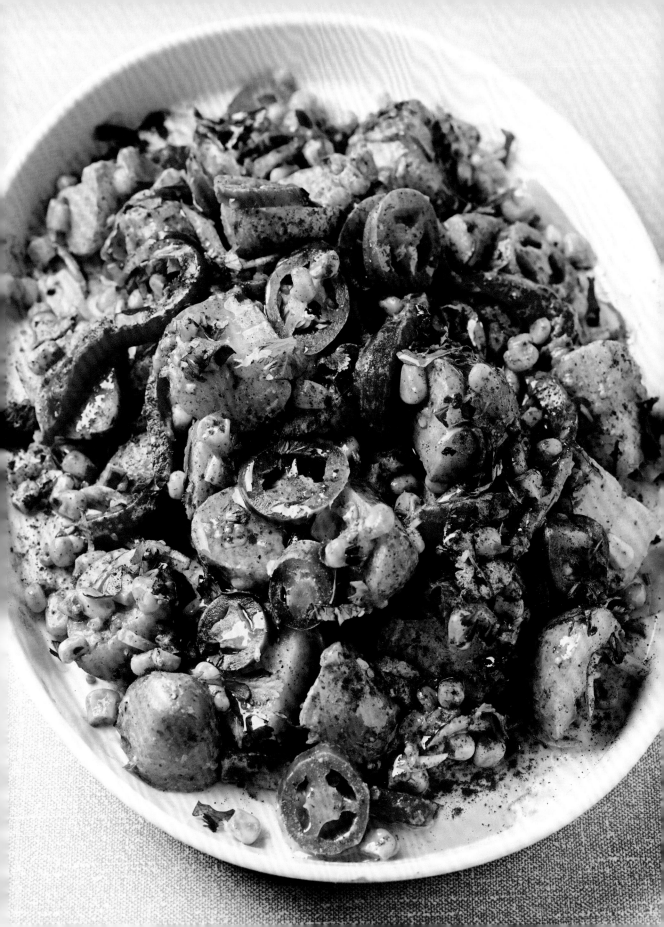

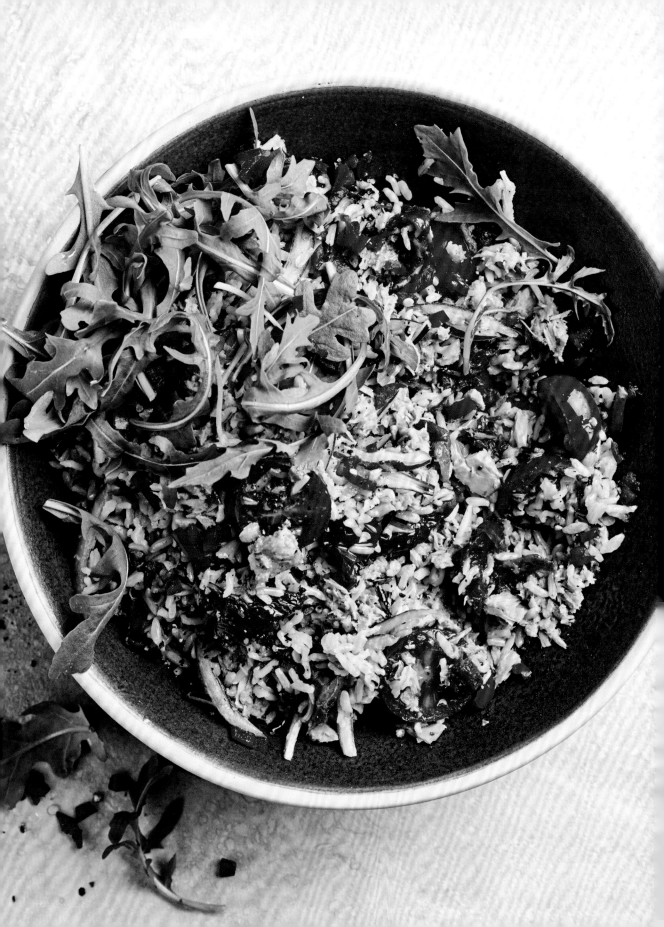

Wild Rice + Tuna Salad

Grab + Go Lunch

Diversity points: 6 / Fibre: 6.7g

2 x 250g (9oz) pouches of pre-cooked wild rice

2 x 160g (5½oz) tins tuna in spring water, drained

200g (7oz) cherry tomatoes, halved

1 small red onion, thinly sliced

8 sun-dried tomatoes, plus a generous tbsp oil from the jar

Juice of 1 lime

1 heaped tsp red chilli powder or 2 finely chopped red chillies

Rocket leaves (optional)

+ Bonus Diversity Points

You can add extra soft herbs like coriander and parsley and serve the salad in romaine lettuce cups. For extra crunch, sprinkle over thinly sliced spring onions and toasted pine nuts and seeds.

Salty tuna, sweet acidic tomatoes and bitter red onions create a marriage made in lunchbox heaven. You can double up the quantities and make enough for four lunchboxes if you prefer. I always try to opt for tuna in spring water instead of brine or sunflower oil for maximum benefit.

1. Heat the rice in the microwave, or according to the instructions on the packet, then tip into a large bowl. Flake the tuna into the rice.

2. Add the cherry tomatoes and sliced red onion to the tuna and rice mixture along with the sun-dried tomatoes (which can be torn roughly) and oil from the jar – this tastes lovely as it is often infused with garlic and tomato juices.

3. To finish the dish, squeeze over the lime juice and add the red chilli, along with a generous handful of rocket leaves (if using). Portion the salad into Tupperware containers and chill in the fridge until ready to eat.

Time Saving Hack
I use wild rice from a pre-cooked pouch to save time, but you can use any other cooked grain here; for example, if you have some pre-cooked spelt or pearl barley ready to use in your fridge.

Coronation Chicken Pasta

Grab + Go
Lunch

Diversity points: 4 / Fibre: 5.2g

250g (9oz) wholewheat fusilli pasta
250g (9oz) cooked chicken, either poached or left over from a roast
250g (9oz) full-fat live Greek yoghurt
½ tsp coarse black pepper
1 tsp ground turmeric
1 tsp ground cumin
½–1 tsp red chilli powder
1 tbsp mango chutney
1 tbsp extra-virgin olive oil
50g (2oz/⅓ cup) raisins
75g (2¾oz/½ cup) toasted almonds (whole or flaked)
Salt, to taste

+ Bonus Diversity Points
Use 250g (9oz) roasted cauliflower for a vegetarian alternative. Add extra spring onions, steamed cauliflower, peas, parsley and chunks of carrot to the pasta. Serve on top of roughly torn cos lettuce leaves.

Coronation chicken is a guilty pleasure of mine. The sweet spicy flavours of the sauce really appeal to my hybrid South Asian-British taste buds. Here I have given coronation chicken the gut-health treatment, with live yoghurt, anti-inflammatory turmeric and fibre-dense toasted almonds featuring against a backdrop of a delicious pasta salad. Delicious, or should I say gut-licious?

1. Start by filling your kettle and boiling it. Tip the pasta into a saucepan, cover with boiling water and add a good pinch of salt. Boil for 8–10 minutes, or until the pasta is cooked through, then drain and set aside to cool.

2. Meanwhile, roughly chop or tear the chicken and place it in a large bowl with the yoghurt, black pepper, turmeric, cumin, red chilli powder, mango chutney and olive oil. Mix everything well and season with salt to taste.

3. Once it has cooled a little, add the cooked pasta to the coronation chicken sauce and stir well to combine, then scatter over the raisins and almonds. Portion into four Tupperware containers and refrigerate until you are ready to eat.

Time Saving Hack
When choosing your pasta, pick one off the shelf that has the shortest cooking time. For fusilli the cooking time can be anything from 6 to 12 minutes!

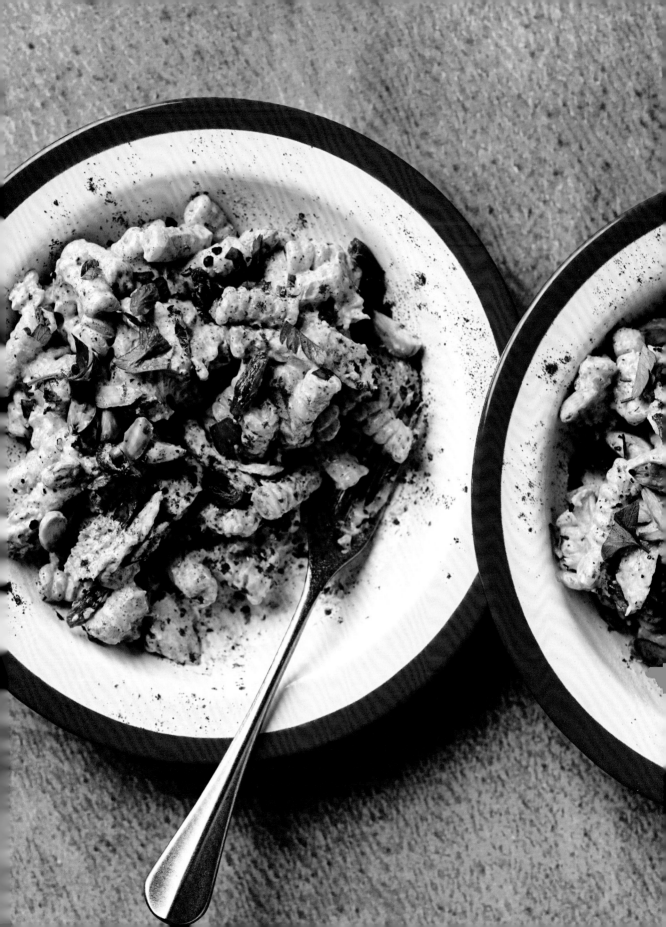

Nutty
Quinoa Salad

Grab + Go
Lunch

Diversity points: 9 / Fibre: 20g

250g (9oz) pre-cooked red and white quinoa (from a pouch)

50g (2oz) bagged spinach, rocket and watercress salad

1 large red apple, diced

200g (7oz) grapes, halved

1 x 400g (14oz) tin green lentils, drained (240g/8½oz drained weight)

Juice of 1 lemon

2 tbsp extra-virgin olive oil

½ tsp black pepper

½ tsp red chilli flakes

Generous handful of toasted whole almonds

Generous handful of pumpkin seeds

Cubes of feta cheese (optional)

Salt, to taste

+ Bonus Diversity Points

Any nuts work well here, either instead of or as well as the almonds. Try walnuts, Brazil nuts or pistachios. You can boost the protein content by adding chickpeas or broad beans and add a herby note with lots of fresh parsley.

This is one of those super-Instagrammable recipes. It is vibrant, nutty, sweet, savoury and very filling: perhaps the very best elements of a good, slightly bougie lunch dish.

1. Heat the quinoa in a microwave, or according to the packet instructions, then tip into a large shallow bowl. Stir to release the steam and cool it slightly.

2. Add the salad leaves, diced apple, grapes and lentils. Squeeze the lemon over the salad (try to get plenty of it on to the apple so that it doesn't brown) and drizzle over the olive oil. Season with salt, black pepper and chilli flakes and toss everything well to combine.

3. Portion into four Tupperware containers and sprinkle over the almonds, pumpkin seeds and feta cubes (if using).

Time Saving Hack
I use quinoa from a pre-cooked pouch and lentils from a tin to save time. You don't have to slice the grapes or chop the almonds, you can leave them whole.

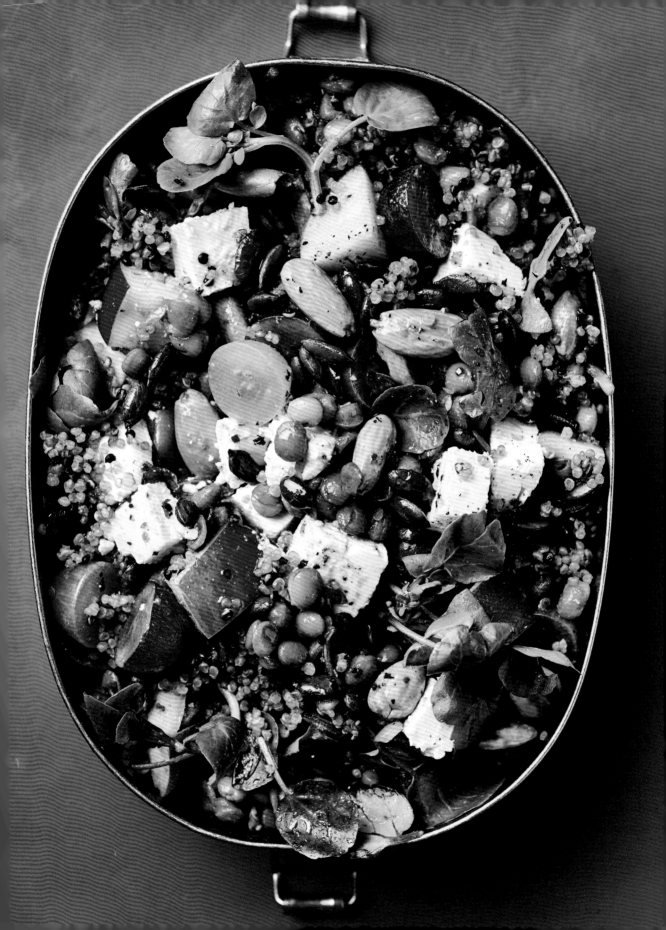

Pesto
Super Grains

Diversity points: 8 / Fibre: 5.8g

250g (9oz) freekeh

75g (2¾oz) jarred roasted peppers, roughly chopped

2 tbsp pitted black olives, roughly chopped

1 ripe tomato, diced

75g (2¾oz) artichokes in brine, roughly chopped

2 tbsp pesto (shop-bought or see page 156)

50g (2oz) baby spinach leaves

2 tbsp toasted pine nuts

120g (4oz) bocconcini mozzarella balls or torn mozzarella (optional)

Salt, to taste

+ Bonus Diversity Points
Use a combination of cooked grains like freekeh, quinoa and pearl barley to experiment with your wholegrains. You can also add any tinned beans or lentils of your choice to the dish.

Freekeh is a fibre-dense Palestinian wheat grain. It tastes quite nutty and keeps its firmness well, which means it maintains its 'bite'. It does need the addition of flavour, and pesto seems to me the perfect pairing.

1. Put the freekeh into a large microwave-safe bowl and top with kettle-hot water to come about 1.5cm (½in) above the freekeh. Cover with a tight lid and microwave for 9 minutes on the highest setting. Carefully remove the lid and stir the grains. If they are a little wet, they will need another minute or two of cooking uncovered. If they are dry, they will need a touch more water followed by a minute or two more cooking. The exact cooking time is difficult to predict due to the age of the freekeh, but 9 minutes seems to work perfectly most of the time for me.

2. While the freekeh is in the microwave combine the peppers, olives, tomato and artichokes in a large bowl with the pesto and baby spinach leaves.

3. Mix in the cooked freekeh, season with salt to taste and stir everything well. You can add a little more olive oil if your pesto is not very oily and the grains seem a bit dry. Top with the pine nuts and mozzarella, portion into four Tupperware containers and keep in the fridge until ready to use.

 Time Saving Hack
Make sure your pantry is stocked with jars of peppers, olives and artichokes so you are always ready to go.

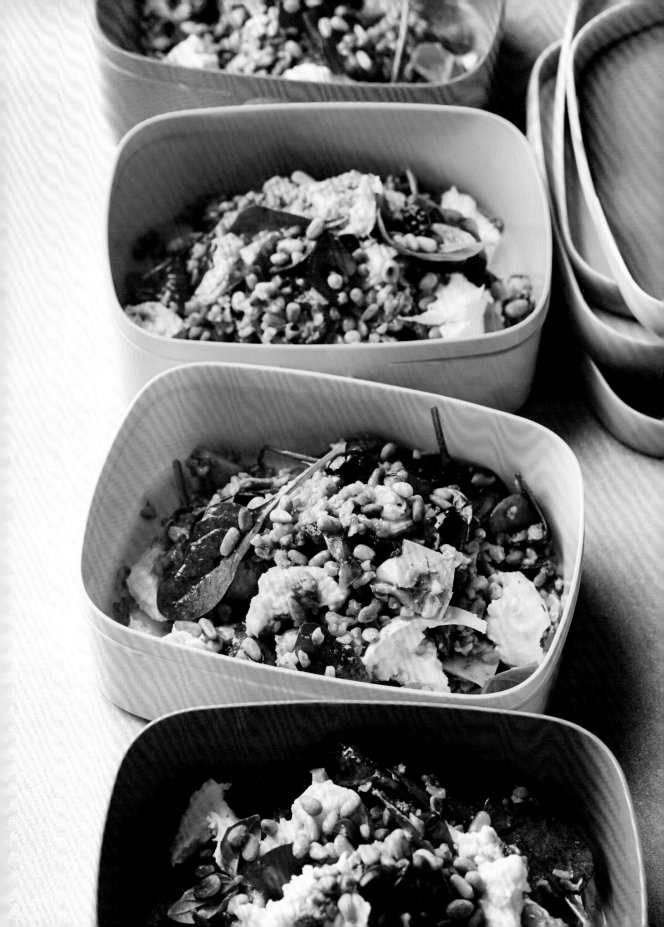

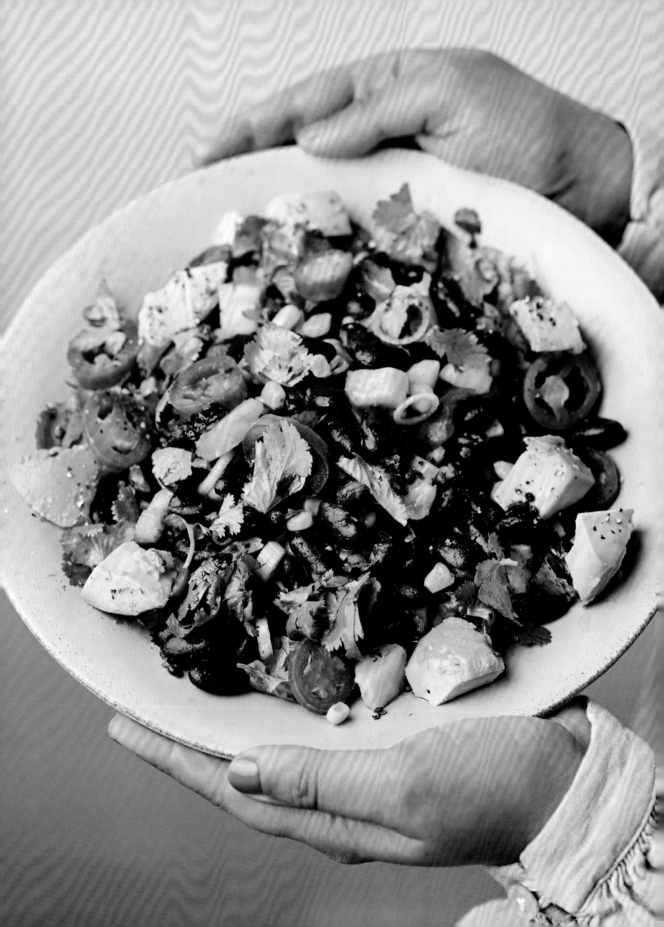

Chipotle Beans

Grab + Go
Lunch

Diversity points: 8 / Fibre: 16g

2 x 400g (14oz) tins kidney beans, drained and rinsed (720g/1½lb drained weight)

1 x 340g (12oz) tin sweetcorn (285g/10oz drained weight)

150g (5oz) mango or the flesh of 1 mango, diced

1 spring onion, thinly sliced

Handful of coriander leaves, roughly chopped

2 heaped tsp chipotle paste

2 tbsp extra-virgin olive oil

Juice of 1 lime

1 tbsp jarred jalapeños, to taste (optional)

Salt, to taste

2 small avocados, spooned into large chunks, to serve (optional)

+ Bonus Diversity Points
You can add tomatoes, pineapple, celery and sliced red onion to the dish.

I've often felt that kidney beans are not given the hype that they deserve. They are so creamy and dense, are packed full of protein and fibre, modest amounts of vitamins and minerals and are so cheap. What's not to love? It is high time we bought kidney beans back in vogue. The chipotle paste should be tasted before adding to the salad as they can vary in strength considerably across brands.

1. Put the drained kidney beans and sweetcorn into a bowl along with the mango, spring onions and coriander. Add the chipotle paste, olive oil and lime juice, season with salt and mix everything well to combine. If you like a bit of heat, stir in the sliced jalapeños.

2. Portion the salad into four Tupperware containers. Serve with ½ avocado per person if you like, for a delicious, creamy contrast to the spiced beans.

Time Saving Hack
Chipotle paste is a real find, giving instant flavour with minimal effort and you can get it in many supermarkets these days. I add it to black beans, marinate chicken and lamb chops with it, and use it in my fajitas and quesadillas. Look for pre-prepared packs of diced mango on supermarket shelves, to save time.

Smacked Cucumbers with Squidgy Chickpeas

Diversity points: 4 / Fibre: 14g

1 cucumber
2 x 400g (14oz) tins chickpeas, drained and rinsed
2 heaped tsp za'atar
2 tbsp extra-virgin olive oil
2 tbsp apple cider vinegar (cloudy)
Large handful of parsley, leaves roughly torn
2 tbsp pomegranate seeds (optional)
Salt, to taste

+ Bonus Diversity Points
Add pistachios, celery and green lentils to the chickpeas and cucumbers. Serve with live probiotic yoghurt for a burst of bacterial goodness.

When I make this dish, I feel like clouds of stress are just dissolving away – there is something very satisfying about smacking a cucumber and squidging some chickpeas. You can use any vinegar you like, but I have opted for apple cider vinegar here on account of its potential probiotic effect. You can use an equal mixture of sesame seeds, dried coriander seeds and dried thyme if you don't have za'atar at home.

1. Slice the cucumber in half lengthways, place the two halves on a chopping board and smash gently with a rolling pin to break the cucumber up into smaller, bite-sized pieces. Place the smashed cucumbers in a bowl.

2. Add the chickpeas to the bowl, firmly pressing them in your hands to break them up as you add them to the bowl.

3. Add the za'atar, extra-virgin olive oil, apple cider vinegar, and torn parsley leaves and stir to combine. Taste and season with salt. Scatter over the pomegranate seeds (if using).

Time Saving Hack
I sometimes mix apple cider vinegar, olive oil and za'atar together to form a dressing. This keeps well in the fridge and I can use it at lunch to dress salad leaves, hard-boiled eggs or even leftover roasted vegetables, like peppers.

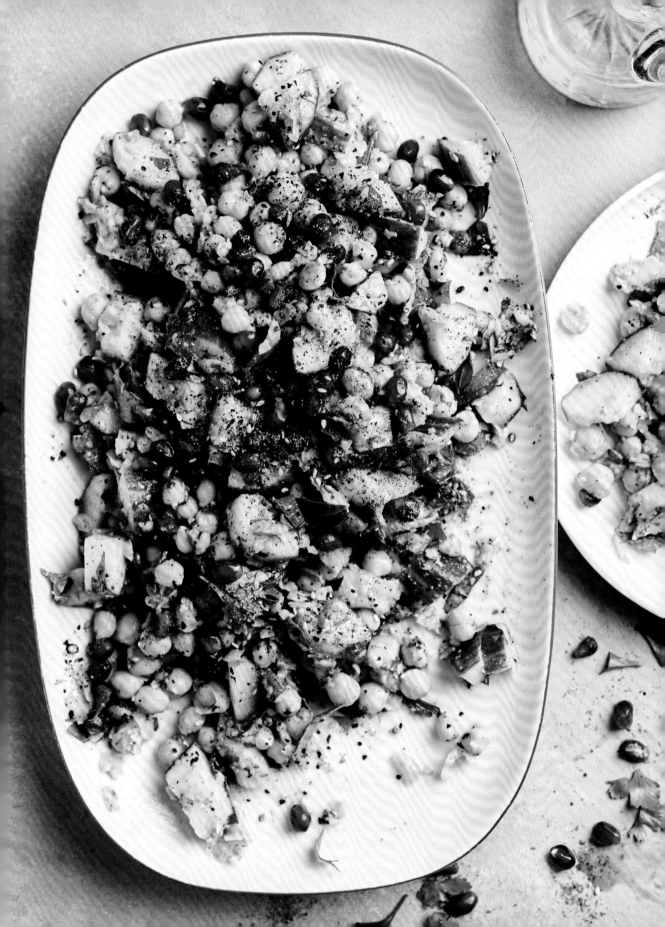

Chilled Beetroot + Kefir Soup

Diversity points: 5 / Fibre: 5.7g

250g (9oz) pre-cooked lightly pickled beetroot (from a vacuum pack)

500ml (17fl oz/2 cups) kefir

½ tsp chilli flakes

Juice of ½ lemon (optional)

Salt, to taste

FOR THE TOPPINGS

200g (7oz) cooked potatoes, diced

¼ cucumber, diced

6 pink radishes, quartered

2 tbsp finely chopped dill

+ Bonus Diversity Points
Spring onions and chives would be a wonderful addition.
You can serve alongside toasted seedy brown bread.

This soup is a cross between a Lithuanian cold beetroot soup called *šaltibarščiai* and the Polish cold beetroot soup *chlodnik*. The addition of potato makes it that bit more substantial and if you want to optimise protein intake, you can also serve it with a hard-boiled egg. It really is the perfect lunch for a summer day, and thankfully, one of the least labour-intensive recipes imaginable.

1. Place the beetroot and half the kefir into a blender along with the chilli flakes and lemon juice. Blitz to a smooth purée and season with salt to taste. Top the soup up with the remaining kefir and stir well before pouring into two serving bowls.

2. Dress the soup with the diced potato, cucumber, radishes and chopped dill. Serve immediately.

Time Saving Hack
Make the beetroot soup up to 2 days in advance and have it ready in the fridge. If you don't have kefir, use buttermilk or full-fat live Greek yoghurt instead.

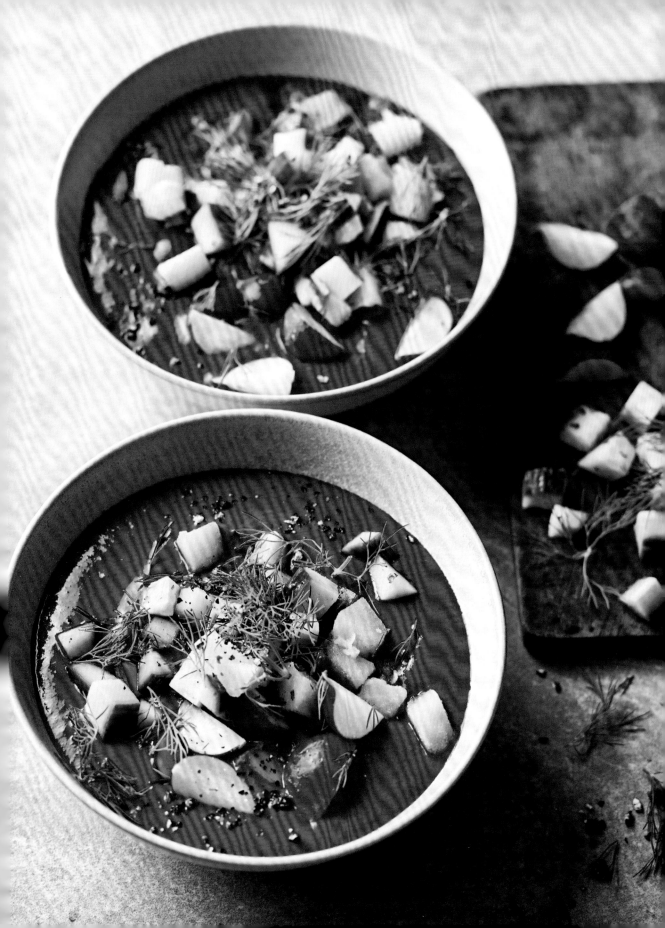

Cheese + Mango Chutney Toastie

Diversity points: 5 / Fibre: 6.2g

75g (3oz) paneer

40g (1½oz) Cheddar cheese

½ tsp ground turmeric

½ tsp black pepper

½ tsp red chilli powder

½ tsp cumin seeds

1 generous tbsp mango chutney

2 slices of sourdough bread

1 tbsp vegetable oil

Handful of baby spinach leaves

1 tomato, thinly sliced

¼ red onion, thinly sliced

+ Bonus Diversity Points
Add chickpeas, green peas and coriander to the cheese mixture.

Is there anything more satisfying than a toastie for lunch? Here I use a combination of paneer and Cheddar cheese to make a wonderful protein-dense filling to this toastie of dreams. The salad ingredients added at the end are essential for crunch and contrast. Tamarind chutney (or more mango chutney) makes a great accompaniment.

1. Grate the paneer and Cheddar into a bowl. Add the turmeric, black pepper, chilli powder and cumin seeds and mix well.

2. Spread the mango chutney over both slices of bread. Top one of the slices with the cheese mixture and top with the other slice of bread (mango chutney side down).

3. Place a non-stick frying pan over a medium heat. Drizzle a little oil into the frying pan and place the toastie into the pan. Fry for 2–3 minutes until golden, then carefully flip it over and cook the other side for 2–3 minutes. Gently prise the sandwich open and stuff it with the spinach leaves, sliced tomato and onion. Serve immediately.

Time Saving Hack
Bring out the toastie machine or panini press lurking at the back of your kitchen cupboard. It will mean that you don't have to spend time flipping the toastie in the frying pan.

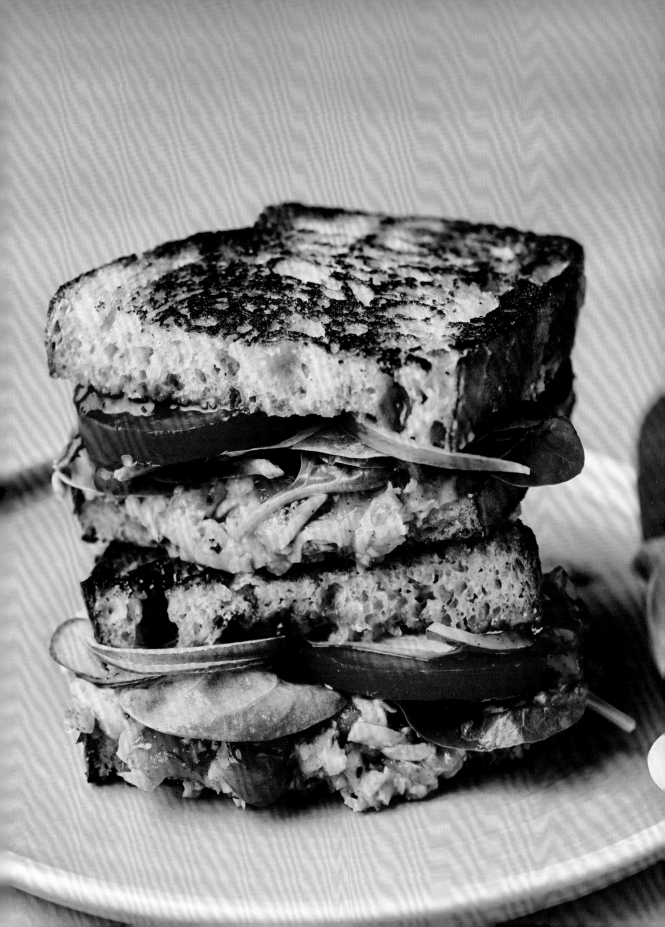

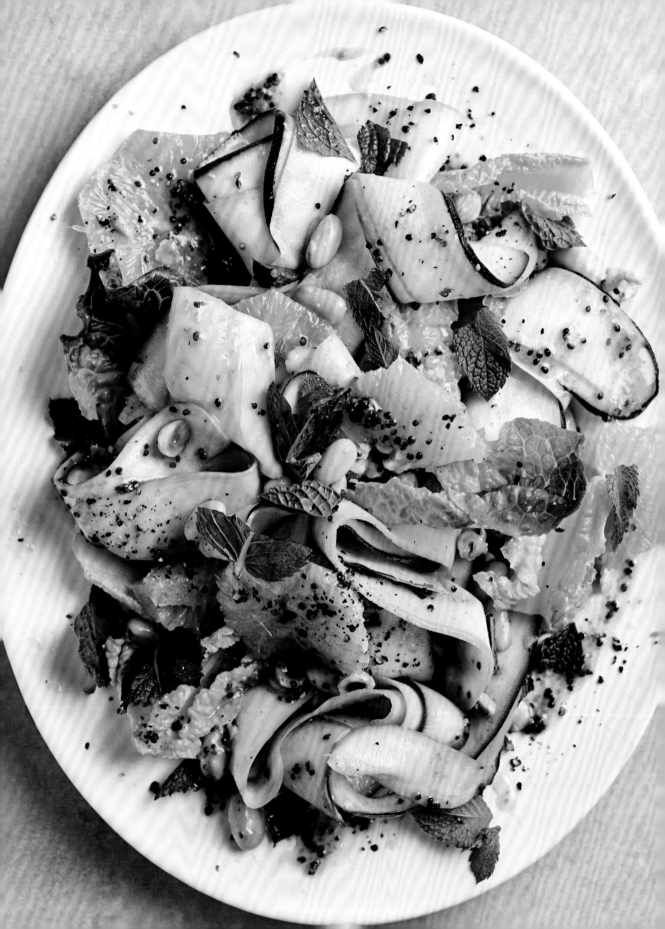

Citrussy Courgette Salad

Lunch at Home

Diversity points: 5 / Fibre: 5.9g

1 courgette (green or yellow)

4–6 cos lettuce leaves

100g (3½oz) tinned cannellini beans

2 small oranges or tangerines

2 tbsp hazelnuts

Handful of mint leaves

Salt, to taste

FOR THE DRESSING

1 tsp honey

1 generous tbsp extra-virgin olive oil

1 tsp Dijon mustard

1 tbsp apple cider vinegar

+ Bonus Diversity Points

Try adding shaved fennel, celeriac or kohlrabi to the salad. You can use other nuts such as pine nuts or peanuts if you wish.

This is such a sophisticated lunch you will hardly believe it takes minutes to prepare. It is the citrus tones that really bring the courgette to life. I use a potato peeler to make courgette ribbons, but you are more than welcome to bring out your spiraliser, or just cut the courgette into rounds.

1. Use a potato peeler to slice the courgette into long ribbons and spread them out on a platter. Tear the lettuce leaves and toss them with the courgette ribbons. Scatter the beans over the courgette and lettuce. Peel the oranges, removing as much white pith as possible, then slice them into rounds. Add these to the salad platter.

2. Mix the honey, olive oil, mustard and apple cider vinegar in a small bowl to make a dressing. Pour this over the salad, season with salt to taste and toss everything well to combine. To serve, scatter over the hazelnuts and a few mint leaves.

Time Saving Hack
Instead of making courgette ribbons, try making quick rounds of courgette in seconds using the slicing blade of your food processor.

CLUB Sandwich:
Carrot Lettuce Under Beet

Lunch at Home

Diversity points: 5 / Fibre: 16g

2 slices of sourdough bread	
½ large carrot	
2 tsp olive oil	
4 pitted black olives, thinly sliced	
Handful of lettuce leaves, chopped	
Handful of parsley leaves	
1 tbsp pesto (shop-bought or see page 156)	
100g (3½oz) pre-cooked vacuum-packed beetroot (can be lightly pickled), sliced	
Pinch of chilli flakes, or to taste	
50g (2oz) goats' cheese, sliced (optional)	

+ Bonus Diversity Points

Add some lentils or chickpeas into your lettuce layer to make it more substantial. Use dark green leaves like spinach, watercress or rocket to further enhance the nutritional content of your CLUB sandwich.

Move over 'chicken and lettuce under bread', there is a new club sandwich in town. This one is altogether more desirable, full of freshness, crunch and heaps of flavour, and most definitely better for your gut. You will be watching the clock at lunchtime, just so that you can tuck in.

1. Lightly toast the sourdough in a toaster.

2. Grate the carrot into a bowl. Squeeze out and discard the excess juice if the carrots are looking a little too watery, then stir in half the olive oil and the sliced black olives. Pile the carrots on to one of the slices of toasted sourdough.

3. Add the chopped lettuce to the same bowl that you prepared the carrots in along with the parsley and pesto, stir to combine, then layer the lettuce over the grated carrots.

4. Finally, add the beetroot, remaining teaspoon of olive oil and chilli flakes to the same bowl and mix together. Layer the beetroot over the lettuce leaves, followed by the sliced goats' cheese (if using).

5. Top with the other slice of toasted bread and press the sandwich down. Slice in half and serve, or wrap and take with you to work.

Time Saving Hack
Using pre-cooked beetroot from a vacuum pack saves time – sometimes I even buy my carrots in pre-grated packs too. If you don't have pesto to hand, use any other dressing of your choice, like a grainy Dijon mustard.

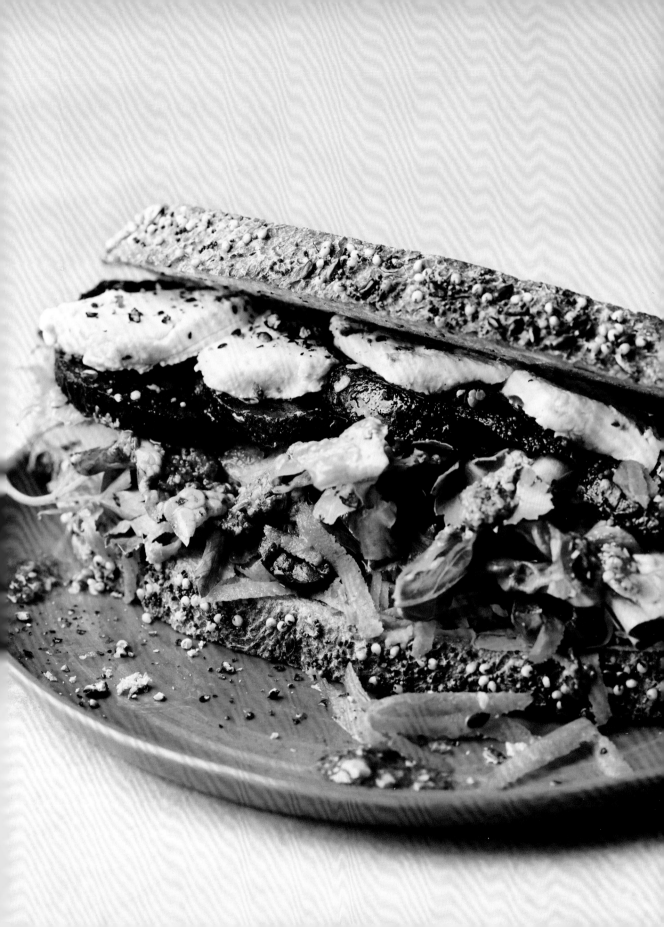

Fridge Raid Bowls from around the World

Diversity points: 5–7

I write this more as a mood board than a prescriptive recipe that you must follow. I want to give you the inspiration to look into your fridge at the random constellation of leftover ingredients and piece them together into a complete bowl of deliciousness, rather like a lunchtime jigsaw puzzle. I have given some ideas from around the world here, but feel free to cross genres when making your own at home.

The key elements that guarantee success are:

1. A grain or starch
2. A few vegetables or pulses
3. A ferment
4. A nut or seed
5. A protein source
6. An acidic dressing to bring everything together

South East Asian Fibre per portion: 5.8g

2 heaped tbsp cooked glass noodles

1 tbsp cooked broccoli

1 tbsp beansprouts

1 tbsp edamame beans

1 heaped tbsp kimchi

1 tsp sesame seeds

1 tbsp cooked prawns or tofu/tempeh

2 tsp rice vinegar

Eastern European Fibre per portion: 14g

2 heaped tbsp cooked pearl barley

1 tbsp cooked beetroot

4–5 pink radishes, halved

1 tbsp wilted kale

1 tbsp pink sauerkraut

1 tbsp pumpkin seeds

1 tbsp cottage cheese

2 tsp apple cider vinegar

Indian Fibre per portion: 6.6g

2 heaped tbsp cooked wild rice

1 tbsp roasted cauliflower

1 tbsp grated carrot

Handful of spinach leaves

1 tbsp full-fat live Greek yoghurt

1 tbsp toasted peanuts

1 tbsp masala chickpeas

Juice of ½ lime

Middle Eastern Fibre per portion: 10g

2 heaped tbsp cooked bulgur wheat

4–5 cherry tomatoes, halved

5cm (2in) chunk of cucumber, diced

1 roasted red pepper

1 tbsp lacto-fermented gherkins

1 tbsp pistachios

1 tbsp hummus

Juice of ¼ lemon

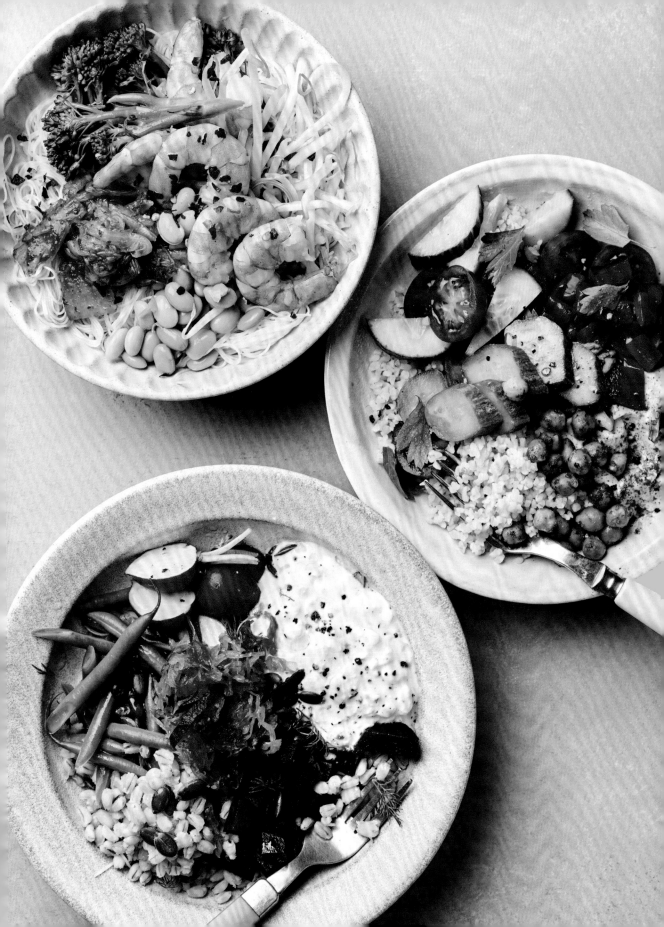

Eggs on Toast

Lunch at Home

Diversity points: 4 / Fibre: 11g

2 slices of sourdough bread

50g (2oz) celery, diced

¼ red onion, diced

½ preserved lemon, diced

50g (2oz) pitted black or green olives, thinly sliced

1 tbsp extra-virgin olive oil

1 tsp harissa paste

2 hard-boiled eggs

Salt, to taste

+ Bonus Diversity Points

Sprinkle cress leaves generously over the egg. For added fibre use rye or sunflower seed bread.

The high protein content of eggs means that they can help us feel fuller for longer. The addition of crunchy celery and onion is a gamechanger, adding much-needed texture to the soft, creamy blandness of boiled eggs.

1. Toast the sourdough bread, either in your toaster or in a frying pan.

2. Put the celery, onion, preserved lemon and olives into a bowl. Stir through the olive oil and harissa, then season to taste with salt.

3. Lay the toasted bread on a plate, then grate the eggs on to the toast. This really does optimise the texture of the dish but if you don't have the energy to do this, then slices of eggs will of course suffice. Spoon the dressing over the eggs and enjoy.

Time Saving Hack
Boil the eggs in the morning so that they are ready to go at lunchtime.

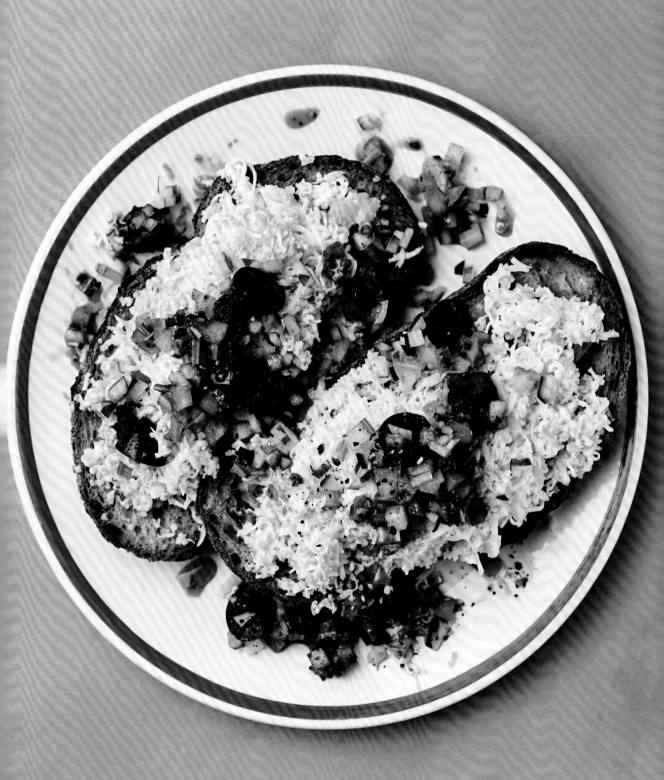

Mushroom Pitta Pizza with Hot Honey Harissa

Lunch at Home

Diversity points: 3 / Fibre: 4.6g

| |
| 1 wholewheat pitta bread (ideally round-shaped) |
| 1 tbsp ricotta cheese |
| 30–50g (1–2oz) goats' cheese, sliced into rounds |
| 2 button mushrooms, thinly sliced |
| 2 tsp extra-virgin olive oil |
| 1 sprig of thyme, leaves picked |
| 1 tsp harissa paste |
| ½ tsp honey |
| 1 tsp roasted hazelnuts |
| Salt and pepper, to taste |

+ Bonus Diversity Points

Add capers, artichokes and rocket leaves to your pizza, as well as a drizzle of the gut-loving pesto on page 156.

Time Saving Hack

Using an air fryer here means your pizza will have a lovely caramelised texture in a really short space of time – it's a bit like having a mini wood-fired oven! If you don't have an air fryer, simply slide the pizza under a conventional grill preheated to medium-high and grill for 5–7 minutes.

I have been making cheat's pizzas for decades. When my parents were out of the house, my sister and I would top naan bread with ketchup and cheese and grill it to perfection to make our own version of a margherita. Uber Eats did not exist in those days! Here I've used a wholewheat pitta bread, which is as free from additives as a non-ultra-processed pizza base. Use this recipe as blueprint; you can use any vegetables you have in your fridge and be as creative as you like. The hot harissa and honey add a welcome contrast and elevate the dish to another level. I use an air fryer for ease, but you can also make this dish in a grill, preheated to medium-high.

1. Spread the ricotta over the pitta bread, leaving a 1cm (½in) border at the edge. Arrange the goats' cheese rounds evenly over the ricotta. Toss the sliced mushrooms in 1 teaspoon of the olive oil, then scatter the mushrooms over the pizza. Scatter the thyme leaves over the mushrooms and season with salt and pepper.

2. Transfer the pizza to your air fryer and air fry at 190°C (375°F) for 5 minutes.

3. Mix the harissa, honey and remaining teaspoon of olive oil together. Drizzle this over the pizza and then continue to air fry for a further 1–2 minutes.

4. Serve immediately with some hazelnuts scattered over the top for maximum enjoyment.

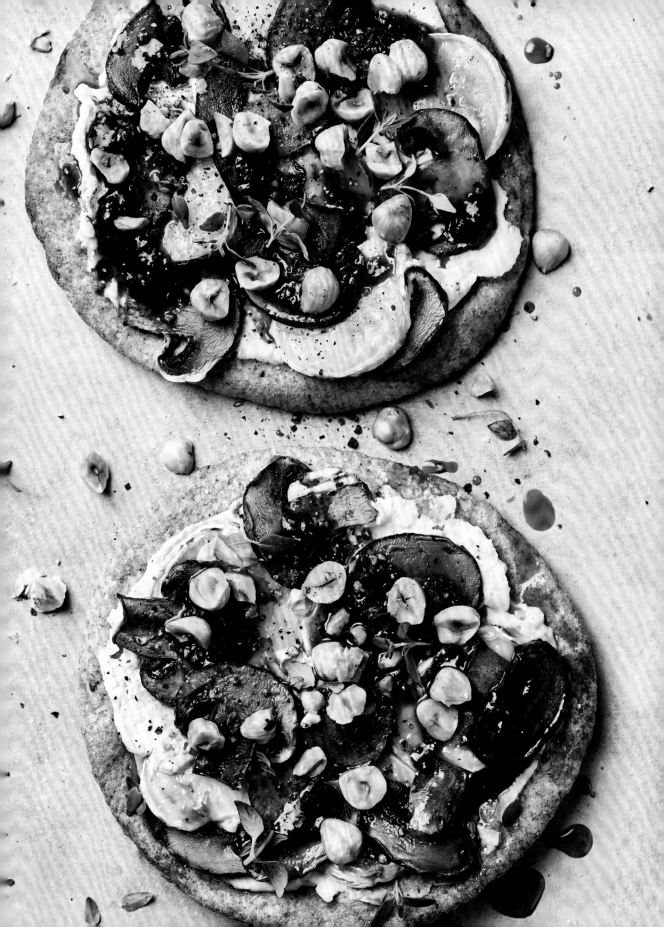

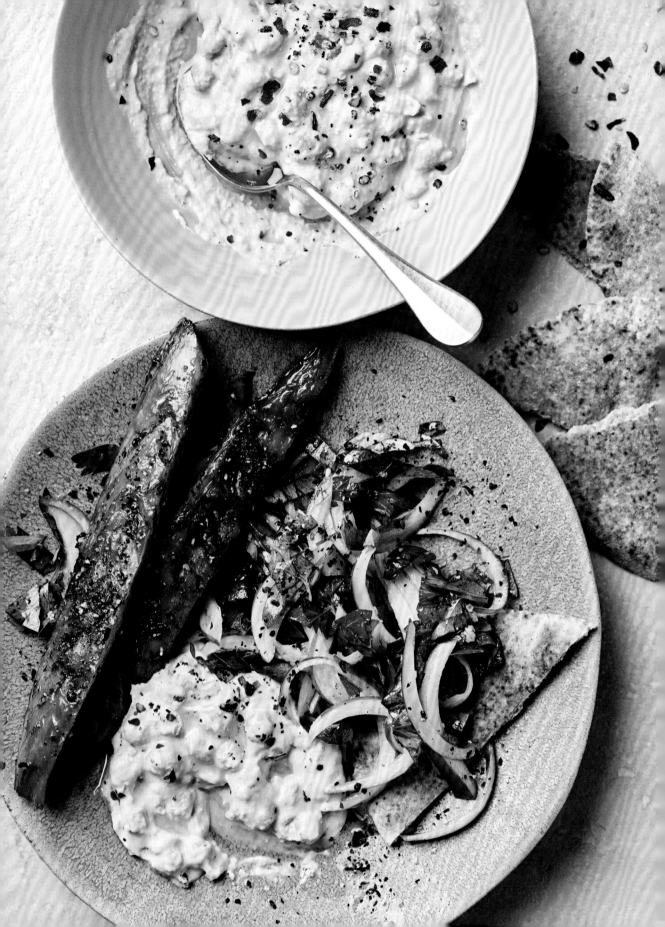

Hummus(ish) with Mackerel + Salad

Lunch at Home

Diversity points: 5 / Fibre: 12g

1 x 400g (14oz) tin chickpeas, drained and rinsed (240g/8½oz drained weight)

2 tbsp full-fat live Greek yoghurt

1 tbsp tahini

½ tsp garlic paste from a jar

½ small red onion, thinly sliced

Handful of parsley leaves, roughly chopped

Juice of ½ lemon

2 peppered smoked mackerel fillets

1 tsp sumac

Red chilli flakes, to taste

1 tbsp extra-virgin olive oil

Salt, to taste

1 toasted wholewheat pitta, to serve

+ Bonus Diversity Points
Serve with sliced ripe tomatoes, toasted pine nuts and sliced cucumber.

This recipe is based on a Middle Eastern dish called *musabaha*, which is essentially a chunky, deconstructed hummus. It makes for a beautiful lunch when paired with a lemony salad and omega-rich mackerel. You can, of course, use any tinned or pre-cooked lentils or beans instead of chickpeas.

1. Add half the chickpeas to a bowl with the yoghurt, tahini and garlic. Use a stick blender to blitz to smooth purée. If you don't have a stick blender just mash everything together with a fork to break down the chickpeas as much as possible. Add the remaining whole chickpeas to the puréed chickpeas and stir well to combine.

2. Put the sliced red onion into a bowl with the chopped parsley and lemon juice, then season with salt and stir to combine. Set aside.

3. Place a small non-stick frying pan over a medium heat. Add the mackerel fillets and cook for just a minute on each side to warm through, then sprinkle over the sumac.

4. Drizzle the chunky hummus with extra-virgin olive oil and finish with a few chilli flakes, then serve with the onion and parsley salad and warmed mackerel. Toasted pitta bread is a wonderful accompaniment.

Time Saving Hack
The great thing about smoked mackerel is that it come pre-cooked in vacuum packs, so is ready to eat whenever you are.

Veg-Tastic Omelette Baguette

Lunch at Home

Diversity points: 6 / Fibre: 7g

3 eggs
½ red/yellow/green pepper, diced
1 tomato, diced
1 green chilli, finely sliced
½ tsp ground turmeric
2 tbsp olive oil
1 medium white baguette (about 180g/6oz)
1 small ripe avocado, halved and stoned
Handful of coriander leaves, roughly torn
Salt, to taste
Hot sauce (optional)

+ Bonus Diversity Points

Add red onions, spring onions and peas to the omelette. Stuff the baguette full of spinach, rocket or watercress leaves.

Time Saving Hack

Have the vegetables that you will use in the omelette diced and ready to go in the fridge. For example, if you are using ½ onion or tomato in a dinner recipe, simply chop the remaining half and keep in a Tupperware container in the fridge, ready for use in your omelette the next day. This is a great way to avoid food waste as well.

A favourite lunch for my husband and me when on the rare occasion we find ourselves working at home together. The egg is merely a vessel for a myriad of delicious vegetables. You can add your favourites: finely chopped broccoli, spring onions and green beans work well if you are going for a greener egg option.

1. Lightly beat the eggs in a bowl and season with a pinch of salt. Add the peppers, tomato and chilli to the eggs along with the turmeric and beat everything well to combine.

2. Heat the olive oil in a non-stick frying over a medium heat. Pour the eggs into the pan and let the mixture cook for a minute or two, then use a spatula to gently lift the cooked egg up, allowing the runny egg to fill the gaps. I like to cook the eggs until the omelette is a golden-brown colour.

3. While the omelette is cooking, halve the baguette lengthways. Scoop the avocado flesh into a small bowl and smash with a fork, then spread it over both cut sides of the baguette.

4. Carefully place the cooked omelette into the avocado-lined baguette and scatter over the coriander leaves. Press the baguette down, cut in half to make two portions and serve hot. Depending on my mood, I like to serve this omelette baguette with a hot sauce.

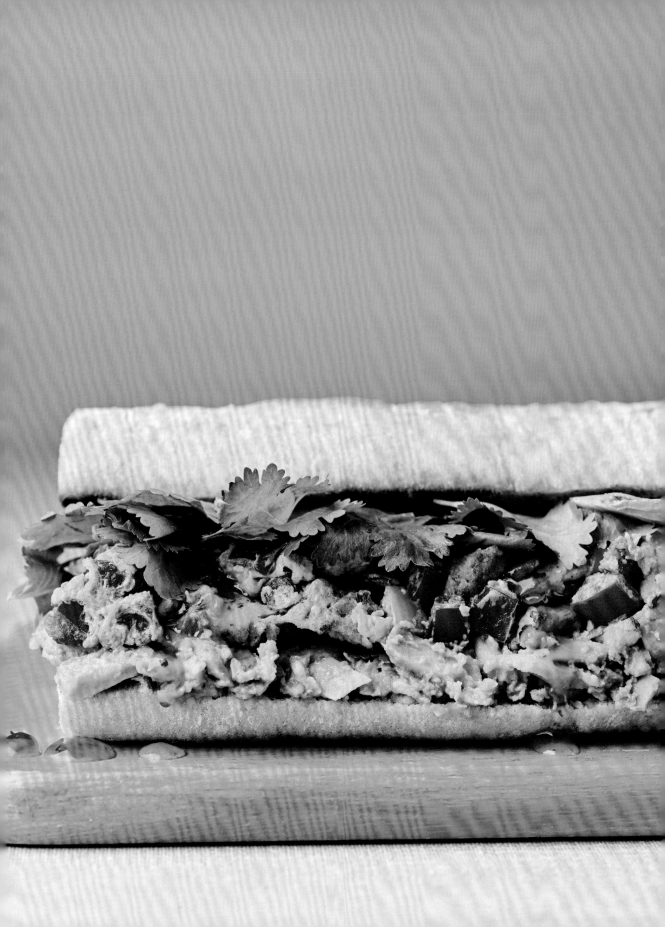

Chop-Chop Salad

A chopped salad is a wonderful thing. You pile all your ingredients on to a board and then use a large knife to chop through the ingredients, forming rough bite-sized chunks. There is no individual chopping of ingredients involved, which makes it a pretty efficient option when it comes to saving time and reducing washing up, not to mention how endlessly versatile a way of using leftovers it will prove to be. I'm not sure why it tastes so much better than a regular salad. I think it must be something to do with the freeform texture and how everything comes together: every bite tasting a bit different to the last.

There are three steps to these recipes:

1. Place the listed ingredients on to a chopping board and cut them roughly into chunks using a large, sharp knife. Transfer the chopped ingredients to a bowl.

2. Add a grain.

3. Dress with the listed ingredients, season with salt to taste and stir well.

Chicken + Herb Tabbouleh

Diversity points: 5
Fibre: 8.8g

STEP 1

100g (3½oz) cooked chicken

Handful of parsley

Handful of coriander

Handful of dill

STEP 2

3 tbsp cooked bulgur wheat

STEP 3

Juice of 1 small lemon

2 generous tbsp olive oil

½ tsp Lebanese allspice

Thai-Inspired Prawn Mango + Mangetout

Diversity points: 6
Fibre: 6.7g

STEP 1

75g (2¾oz) cooked prawns

100g (3½oz) mango pieces

75g (2¾oz) mangetout

2 baby cucumbers

Large handful of coriander

STEP 2

3 tbsp cooked quinoa

STEP 3

1 tbsp fish sauce

Juice of 1 lime

1 green chilli, thinly sliced

1 tsp honey

Smoked Salmon, Potatoes + Eggs

Diversity points: 4
Fibre: 5.6g

STEP 1

6 cooked baby new potatoes

1 hard-boiled egg

75g (2¾oz) smoked salmon

Handful of chives

2 green cabbage leaves

4 cornichons

STEP 2

2 tbsp cooked buckwheat or faro

STEP 3

2 tbsp live yoghurt

1 heaped tsp horseradish sauce

Juice of ½ lemon

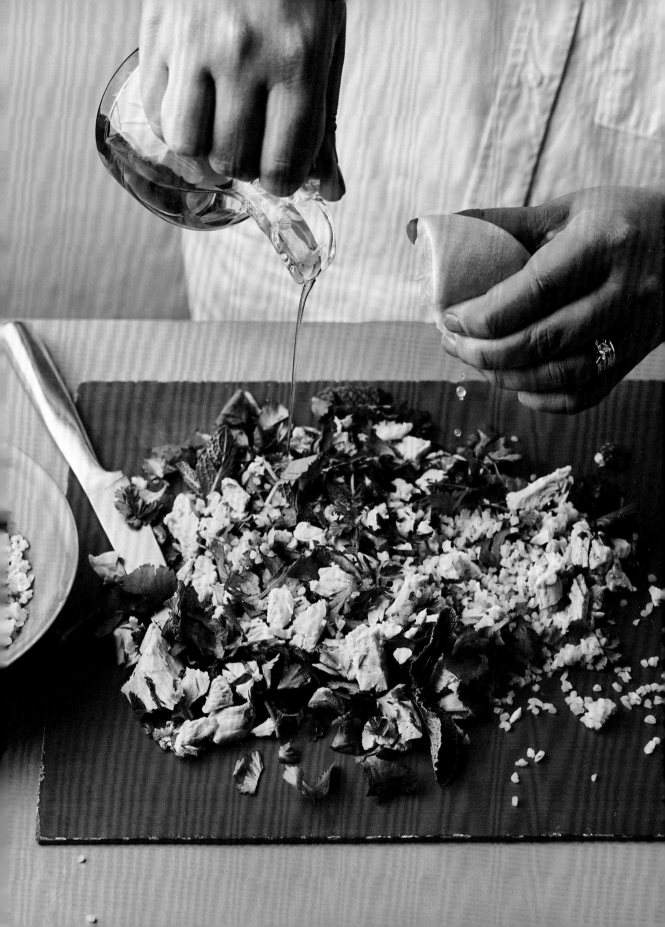

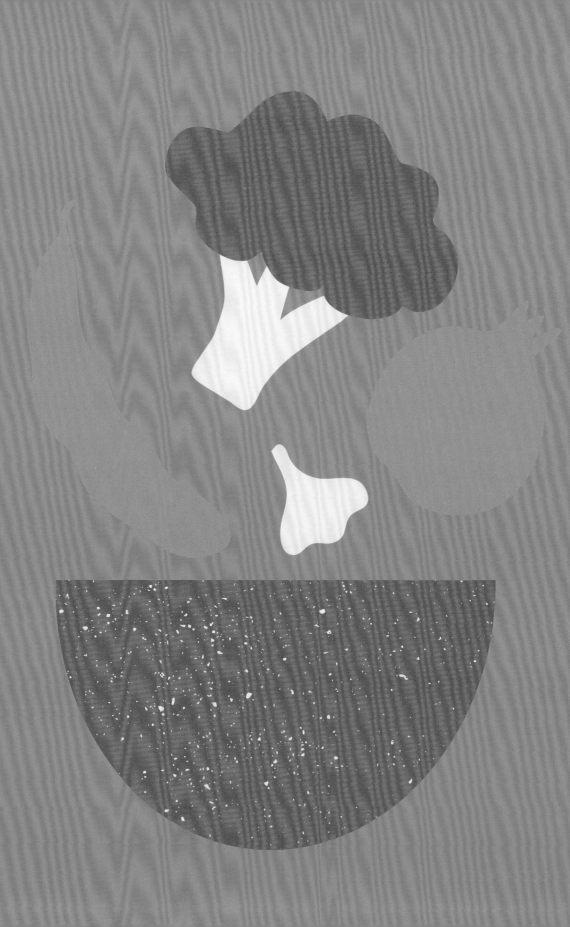

Winner Winner Quick Dinner

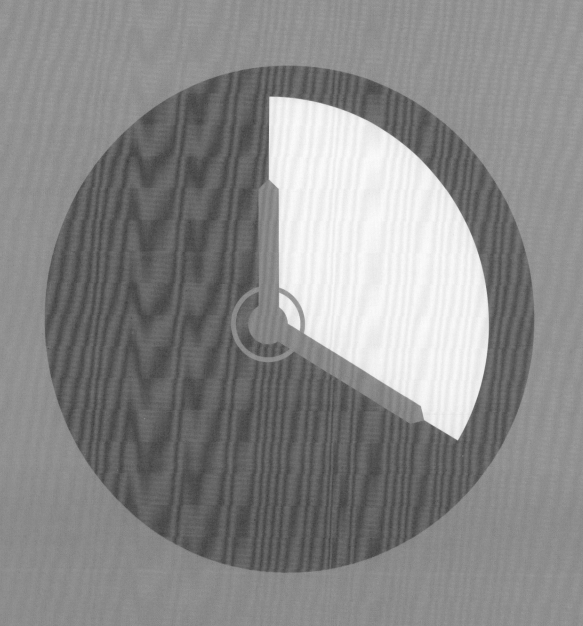

For many people one of the most tedious things about being an adult is having to come up with an idea for dinner, shopping for the ingredients, cooking and then cleaning up. And then repeating the whole process night after night for the foreseeable future. If you've ever felt that unending pressure to think of something for dinner that's a) healthy, b) but also won't break the bank, c) won't dirty too many pans and d) won't be immediately snubbed by the kids, then this chapter is for you.

For me, preparing dinner has lately become an oasis of calm amid the chaos that is family life. Here, I get twenty minutes (if I'm lucky) of uninterrupted time (if I'm lucky) where I can be my authentic self and find some semblance of peace (if I'm lucky). Clinking pots and pans, chopping and stirring, feeling and smelling the ingredients to create two or three platefuls of delicious, nutritious food is for me quite meditative, almost like culinary tai chi or tending a zen garden. Cultivating this mindset didn't come overnight, but now that I have it I really do value it.

This chapter is the largest in this book because of the huge impact that dinner can have on our health, and because it is where I feel most people can make positive changes to their gut health. While breakfast and lunch have immense value, it's clear that dinner is the keynote speaker at the meal conference, the main event.

The recipes in this chapter function as your very own gut health cheat cards; not only do they pack a real punch in flavour, but they also contain a range of ingredients that will bring your gut bacteria back to optimal operations. The influences are global, from the Far East to Italy, South America to Africa; my hope is that this will encourage you to increase the diversity and variety of your evening menus, making it easier for you to 'eat the rainbow'.

I have also designed these recipes with our already-stretched budgets in mind, so I've tried to use inexpensive ingredients to give you the maximum benefit for each pound you hand over at the checkout.

Although meat and fish feature in these recipes, it is the vegetables that I want to highlight as the true stars of many of these dishes. Whole grains feature heavily, as do tinned legumes and pulses. The recipes are versatile and many are presented as a foundation upon which you can build your own personal 'dish-de-la-resistance'. I encourage all readers to tailor the recipes to your own tastes, and to use what you have in your freezer and store cupboard to make gut-healthy swaps.

The recipes in this chapter are divided into three 'mini' chapters: Fakeaways, Lighter Suppers and Comforting Dinners.

Fakeaways

These are gut-friendly recipes inspired by takeaway classics. Let's not beat around the bush: everyone loves an occasional takeaway. The mixture of carbs, salt, sugar, MSG and fat, all bundled up into energy-dense, effort-free deliciousness is often hard to resist. But within that deliciousness also lies their danger. I know people who have gone as far as deleting the delivery apps from their phone and hiding their devices at dinner time to avoid the constant temptation.

Here's where my recipes come in. Not only are they (if I may say so myself) as tasty as any takeaway, but they also come without all the extra additives, salt and other nasties so often found in ultra-processed takeaway food. These 'fakeaway' dishes are designed so that you can prepare them in less time than it takes for the delivery driver to get to your house with the twenty nuggets and chips meal. Now, I'm not saying don't ever buy a takeaway again; they can be fun, enjoyable and sometimes necessary. Instead I want to show you how easy the alternatives can be. So, put takeaways back where they belong, as a once-in-a-while treat rather than a regular dinner habit.

Light Suppers

To be honest, the distinction between a 'light' meal and a 'heavy' one is a bit arbitrary. Here I've included wholesome meals that will still make you feel full, ideal for when the mood calls for bright, airy freshness and a light touch. I tend to opt for these recipes when I have had a big lunch or a late snack but still have a bit of space left for dinner. The recipes featured in this chapter can also double up as lunch recipes, which is rather handy.

Comforting Dinners

It is a fallacy that gut-healthy eating can't be warm and comforting. The recipes in this section are food for your soul as well as your gut. They do something for the emotional being within us, lifting us further and further away from our troubles with each mouthful. There's no denying that good food contributes to good mood, and the only thing I hope you enjoy more than cooking these recipes is eating them.

Supporting your digestive health through your dinner choices is not hard, but it is a learned skill; like any skill it takes time to know which ingredients or dishes will contribute most to your gut health. To start with, here are a few guiding comments to bear in mind before I send you on your way.

1. Don't try to completely cut out certain food groups, it is not sustainable in the long term. As with everything, moderation is key.

2. Don't leave dinner too late. Leaving plenty of time between dinner and bedtime will reduce or even prevent reflux, benefit your metabolism, and give your gut bacteria some much-needed rest time.

3. Examine the elements of these recipes and in light of your newfound knowledge about gut-healthy eating. Try to identify what exactly makes these recipes good for you. Are their lots of prebiotics or probiotics included? Is the fibre count high? Is the diversity score high?

4. Finally, the person who does the cooking doesn't do the dishes. Non-negotiable.

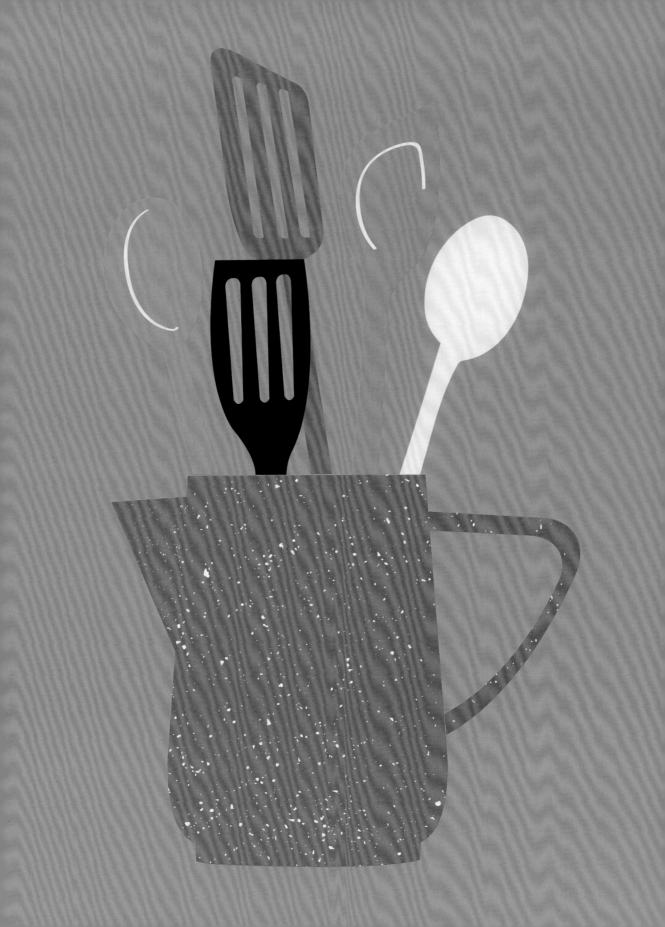

Shawarma Shrooms, Green Sauce + Crispy Pitta

Diversity points: 5 / Fibre: 9.8g

750g (1lb 10oz) mushrooms, roughly chopped or torn

2 tbsp shawarma seasoning

4 generous tbsp vegetable oil

½ small red cabbage, thinly sliced

Juice of ½ lemon

4 wholewheat pittas or other flatbreads, to serve

FOR THE GREEN SAUCE

60g (2½oz) parsley

3 heaped tbsp tahini

2 heaped tbsp full-fat live Greek yoghurt

Salt, to taste

+ Bonus Diversity Points
Serve with lacto-fermented pickles and extra salad (onions, cucumbers, tomatoes) dressed with sumac.

Time Saving Hack
Ready-made shawarma seasoning can be found in many shops, and will save you having to measure out individual spices. If you can't find it, use baharat spice mix or a mixture of black pepper, ground cumin, coriander seeds and garlic granules. If you have an air fryer the mushrooms will cook in 7–9 minutes at 200°C (400°F).

When all you can think of is a doner kebab, this is the perfect gut-healthy treat. It has all the familiarity of a takeaway in its flavour and texture profile but is fundamentally a healthy vegetarian dinner dish. It's just waiting to become your new go-to recipe.

1. Put the mushrooms into a bowl, sprinkle over the shawarma seasoning and drizzle over 2 tablespoons of the vegetable oil. Mix well so that the seasoning has coated all the mushrooms.

2. To make the sauce, add the parsley, tahini and yoghurt to a blender along with a few tablespoons of kettle-hot water. Blend to a smooth green purée, then season with salt to taste and set aside.

3. Squeeze the lemon half over the sliced red cabbage, season with salt to taste and set aside. Place the pitta breads or flatbreads in your toaster (or in a dry frying pan on the hob) and allow them to brown slightly.

4. While the bread is toasting, heat a tablespoon of vegetable oil in a wok over a very high heat. When the oil is smoking hot, add the mushrooms and stir-fry for 3–4 minutes until they cook through and are a deep golden-brown colour. If the oil in the wok isn't hot enough the mushrooms will stew and you won't achieve the desired colour.

5. To serve, roughly tear the pitta or flatbread and arrange over four plates. Top with the mushrooms, red cabbage and lashings of the green tahini sauce.

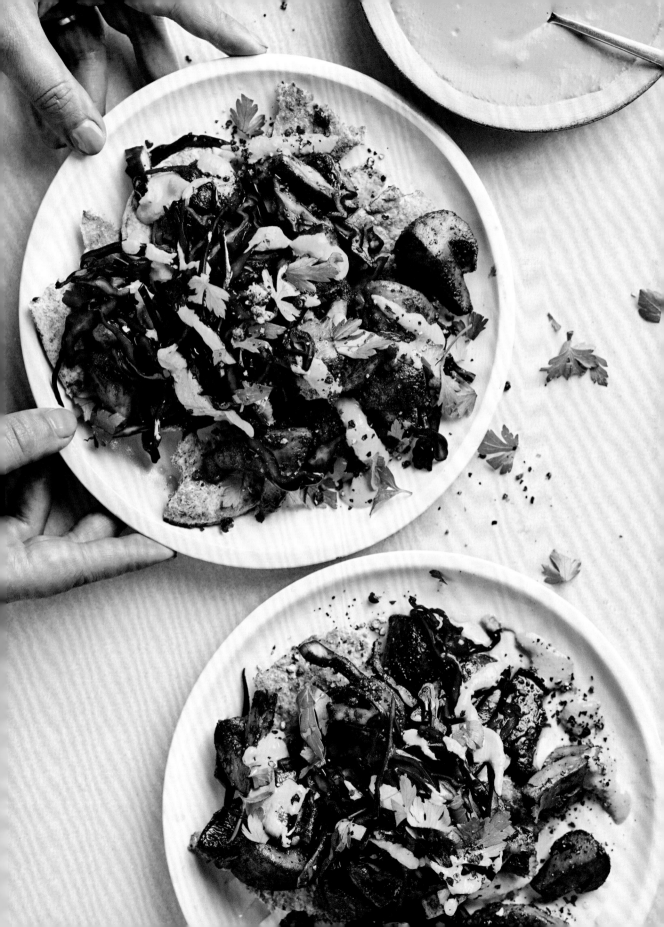

Roasted Cauliflower Korma

Diversity points: 6 / Fibre: 14g

800g (1lb 12oz) cauliflower, cut into florets

2 tsp ground turmeric

2 tbsp olive oil

100ml (2½fl oz/scant ½ cup) kettle-hot water

FOR THE SAUCE

2 x 400ml (14fl oz) tins coconut milk

4 tbsp crispy fried onions

150g (5oz/1¼ cups) ground almonds

1 tsp ground turmeric

2 tsp cumin seeds

2 tsp red chilli flakes

2 tsp garam masala

2 heaped tsp garlic paste

2 heaped tsp ginger paste

TO SERVE

Handful of almonds, roughly chopped

Coriander leaves, roughly torn/chopped

4 naan bread

+ Bonus Diversity Points

Try this recipe with any brassicas of your choice, e.g. cabbage and broccoli florets.

Time Saving Hack

Crispy fried onions impart colour and flavour to the dish and I often use them to save the 10 minutes it takes to chop and brown an onion on the stove. When buying the onions and naan in the shops, try to pick versions which are not full of additives and preservatives or palm oil.

There are moments in life where nothing but a korma will suffice, and for those moments there is this recipe. There are so many ways I cheat in this recipe. From buying bags of pre-cut cauliflower florets to using crisp fried onions from a packet and garlic and ginger from a jar.

1. Put the cauliflower florets into a bowl, dust with the turmeric and drizzle over the extra-virgin olive oil. Toss well together and transfer to the air fryer for 10–12 minutes at 200°C (400°F). (If you are not using an air fryer, roast the cauliflower in an oven preheated to 200°C fan/220°C/gas mark 7 for 12–15 minutes.) Give the contents of the air fryer a shake halfway through so that the heat distributes evenly. You are looking for the cauliflower to still have a little bit of a crispness to it, but for many of the edges to be charred and golden.

2. While the cauliflower is roasting, blitz all the ingredients for the sauce together in a blender to make a thick purée. Pour this purée into a wide saucepan, add the water and simmer over a low-medium heat for 5–6 minutes until the oil starts splitting from the sauce and the raw taste has gone; the colour will also deepen a little. You can adjust the consistency and make the sauce looser with hot water if you prefer, but I like it quite thick.

3. To serve, pour this sauce into a dish and top with the roasted cauliflower florets, then scatter over the chopped almonds and coriander. I like to serve alongside some quick toasted/microwave-heated naan breads.

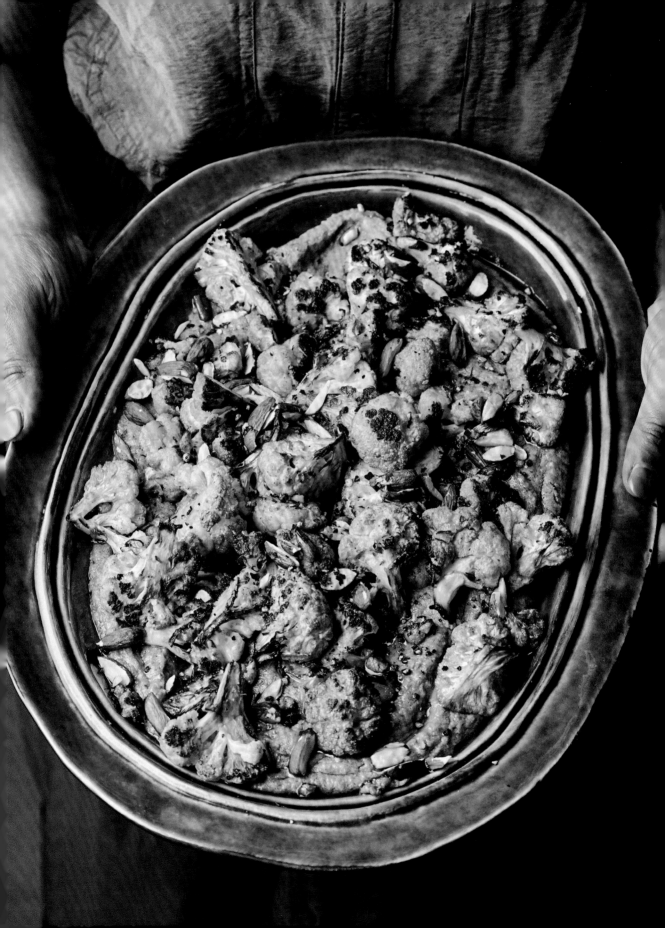

Prawn Tacos with Gut-Loving Relish

Fakeaways

Diversity points: 6 / Fibre: 8.2g

400g (14oz) jumbo raw peeled prawns (**not frozen**)

1 tsp smoked paprika

½ tsp red chilli powder

1 x 400g (14oz) tin black beans, drained

8 corn and wheat tortillas (30cm/12in in diameter)

1 tbsp vegetable oil

¼ red cabbage, thinly sliced

FOR THE RELISH

200g (7oz) pineapple chunks, diced

2 kiwi fruits, peeled and diced

Juice of ½ lime

½ tsp smoked paprika

Salt, to taste

TO SERVE (OPTIONAL)

Soured cream

Jalapeños from a jar

Chopped coriander

+ Bonus Diversity Points

Serve with avocado and thinly sliced red onions pickled in apple cider vinegar.

A great little hack for if you are constipated is to eat a couple of kiwi fruit a day. They are full of fibre and an enzyme called actinidin, which helps soften things for many people. The trouble is that it can get quite boring eating plain kiwi fruit every day. These tacos are topped with a delicious sweet and tart pineapple and kiwi relish so you can sneak in the kiwi with your dinner.

1. Place the prawns in a bowl and sprinkle over the paprika and chilli powder. Stir to combine well.

2. To make the relish, combine all the ingredients in a bowl and mix to combine, then taste and adjust the seasoning.

3. Rinse the drained black beans through with kettle-hot water to warm them through. Heat up your tortillas, either in the microwave or in a large flat frying pan. Wrap them in a clean tea towel to keep warm.

4. Place a non-stick frying pan over a high heat and pour in the vegetable oil. When the pan is hot but not yet smoking, add the prawns and cook them quickly so that they get a nice colour. They will take just 2–3 minutes to cook through.

5. To serve, pile the warm tortillas with black beans, red cabbage, prawns and the pineapple and kiwi relish. Top with soured cream, jalapeños and chopped coriander, if you like.

Time Saving Hack
I sometimes buy pots of fresh pineapple chunks – you'll often find it discounted in the supermarket towards the end of the day. You can also use frozen (and defrosted) or tinned pineapple (in juice, not syrup) here as well.

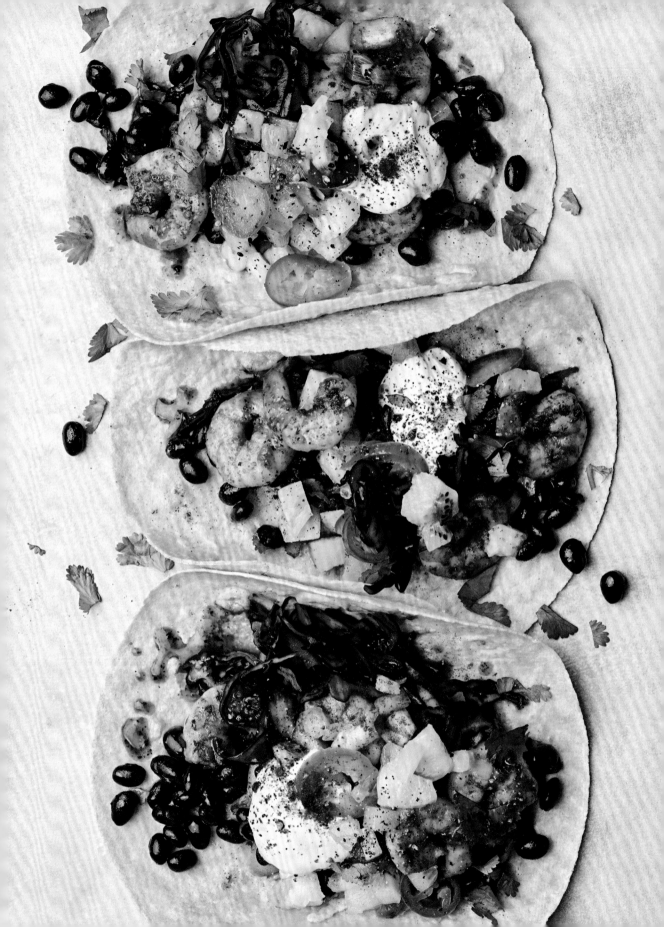

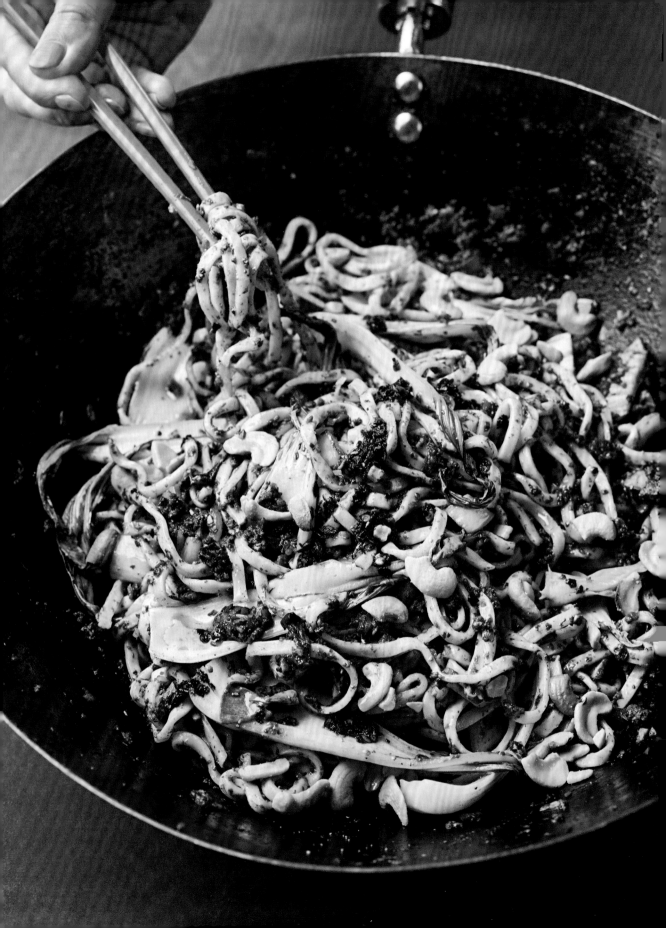

Mushroom Dan Dan

Diversity points: 5 / Fibre: 4.2g

300g (10oz) button mushrooms

1 x 225g (8oz) tin sliced water chestnuts (140g/4½oz drained weight)

2 tsp garlic paste

3 tbsp dark soy sauce

2 tbsp hoisin sauce

2 tbsp rice wine vinegar

1-2 tsp chiu chow chilli oil, plus a drizzle to serve

1 heaped tsp Chinese five-spice

2 tbsp vegetable oil

3–4 x 150g (5oz) packs of vacuum-packed, pre-cooked udon noodles

Large handful of toasted cashews

+ Bonus Diversity Points

Add some thinly sliced pak choi or peppers and onions to the wok with the mushroom and water chestnut mixture. Alternatively, steam some pak choi in the microwave and serve dressed with a teaspoon of sesame oil and a few sesame seeds as a quick side dish.

A deeply spiced and umami noodle dish. I use ready-to-use udon noodles here, but you can use any noodles you love. Dan Dan noodles are usually made with red meat, like beef, but the combination of earthy mushrooms and crunchy water chestnuts is really quite pleasing – and substantially cheaper.

1. Put the button mushrooms into a food processor along with the water chestnuts and garlic paste. Blitz until the texture loosely resembles grains of rice.

2. Combine the soy sauce, hoisin sauce, rice wine vinegar, chilli oil and five-spice in a small bowl with a few tablespoons of water and stir well to combine. This is your stir-fry sauce.

3. Heat the vegetable oil in a wok over a high heat; when hot, add the mushroom and water chestnut mixture and cook through for about 2 minutes before adding the stir-fry sauce and the cooked udon noodles.

4. Add a further few splashes of water and stir everything well to combine. After another minute or two of cooking the noodles will be coated in a silky sauce and ready to serve. I like to scatter over toasted cashews and sometimes (mood dependant) extra chilli oil.

Time Saving Hack
I appreciate that using pre-cooked noodles may be a step too far for some, and by all means, boil your own from scratch. But on very busy evenings, there is something incredibly comforting about having these noodles sitting ready in the pantry.

Thai Green Curry
Noodle Broth

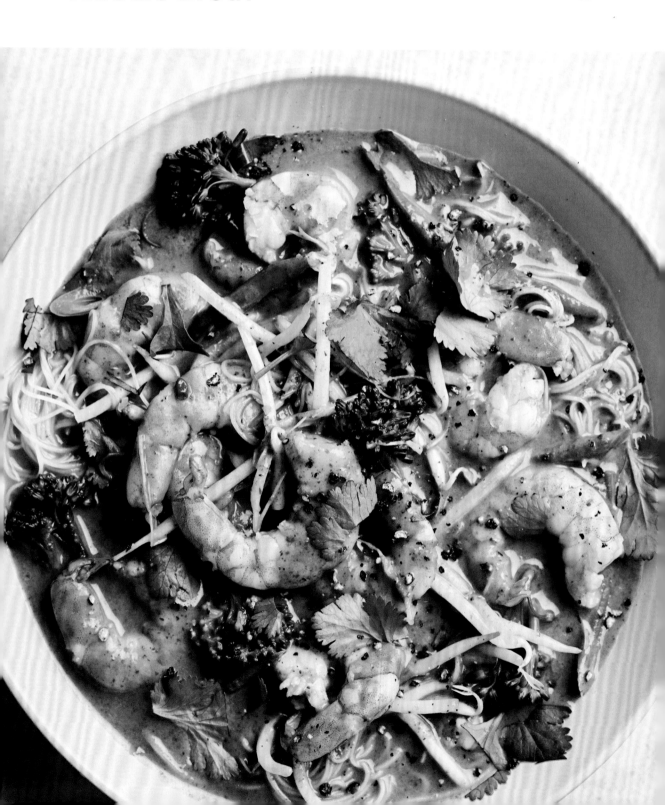

Diversity points: 7 / Fibre: 12g

4 heaped tbsp green curry paste

2 x 400ml (14fl oz) tins full-fat coconut milk

2 tbsp fish sauce

2 tsp brown sugar

4 large handfuls of spinach leaves

Juice of 2 limes

200g (7oz) green beans

200g (7oz) Tenderstem broccoli

4 nests of rice noodles

150g (5oz) beansprouts

240g (8½oz) cooked peeled prawns

Chopped coriander (optional)

Salt, to taste

+ Bonus Diversity Points
Experiment with the greens in this the dish – try adding
frozen peas and edamame beans to your green curry soup.

Time Saving Hack
Use Thai red curry paste instead of green for a
change. I use rice noodles as they take no time to
make but you can use any pre-cooked noodles you
like, such as udon or egg noodles.

This recipe lives or dies by the quality of the green curry paste. There are so many different varieties available these days. I try to choose one that is not laden with too many extra additives and preservatives, and that tastes quite pungent. There are even some really good organic, non-ultra-processed curry pastes available online so it's well worth seeking out your favourite one if you haven't got the time to make your own... and quite frankly, who does these days?

1. Start by putting a kettle of water on to boil.

2. Put the green curry paste, coconut milk, fish sauce and brown sugar into a saucepan and place over a medium heat. Simmer for a few minutes until the mixture has heated through and is bubbling away. Add the spinach and juice of half a lime and cook just until the spinach has wilted down.

3. Use a stick blender to blend the sauce to a smooth purée – the spinach will give it a vivid green colour. (Don't worry if you don't have a stick blender, this is not an essential step.) If you prefer a thinner, more soupy sauce, you can adjust to your desired consistency with kettle-hot water. Season with salt to taste, bearing in mind that many green curry pastes have salt added already.

4. Roughly chop the green beans and broccoli and place in a microwave-safe bowl with a splash of water. Microwave on high for 3 minutes.

5. Place the rice noodle nests in a heatproof bowl and pour kettle-hot water over them. Leave to steep for 3 minutes before draining in a sieve.

6. To assemble the noodle soup, place a handful of noodles in the bottom of each bowl and top with the prawns, green beans, broccoli and beansprouts. Poor over the green curry sauce and serve immediately, scattered with some chopped coriander, if you have it.

Express Paneer Jalfrezi Wraps

SERVES 4

Diversity points: 5 / Fibre: 3.2g

400g (14oz) paneer

1 red pepper, cut into large chunks

1 heaped tbsp jalfrezi paste

1 tbsp olive oil

4 flatbreads/naan breads

4 tbsp full-fat live Greek yoghurt

Handful of rocket leaves

FOR THE MANGO AND CUCUMBER SALAD

200g (7oz) mango, diced

5cm (2in) piece of cucumber, diced

½ tsp cumin (either use ground cumin or lightly crushed cumin seeds)

Juice of ½ lemon

½ tsp chilli flakes

Salt, to taste

+ Bonus Diversity Points

Add tomatoes, onions and coriander leaves to the wraps to boost the salad content.

Paneer is such a fantastic alternative to meat. It takes far less time to cook and is a sponge for any strong flavours. So when the craving for a takeaway strikes, why not try these fantastic spicy jalfrezi-inspired paneer wraps? Use your favourite ready-made jalfrezi paste but do take time to check the ingredients lists; there are quite a few on the market now that are free from additives and preservatives, usually made from mix of dry spices suspended in oil.

1. Slice the block of paneer into chunks that roughly resemble the size and shape of fishfingers. Add these to a bowl along with the red pepper, jalfrezi paste and olive oil. Mix well to combine. Transfer to an air fryer and roast at 200°C (400°F) for 7 minutes, turning the paneer and peppers over halfway through. If you don't have an air fryer, you can fry the paneer and peppers in a non-stick frying pan over a high heat for 6–7 minutes. You are looking for charred, darkened edges.

2. Put the mango and cucumber into a small bowl and season with the cumin, lemon juice, chilli flakes and salt and set aside.

3. Heat the flatbreads in a dry frying pan or in the microwave. Spread a tablespoon of Greek yoghurt over each flatbread and top with the rocket, jalfrezi paneer and mango and cucumber salad. Roll into wraps and serve immediately.

Time Saving Hack

Instead of raiding the spice cupboard, use a shop bought spice paste. If you don't have jalfrezi paste at home, you can use harissa paste in this recipe instead.

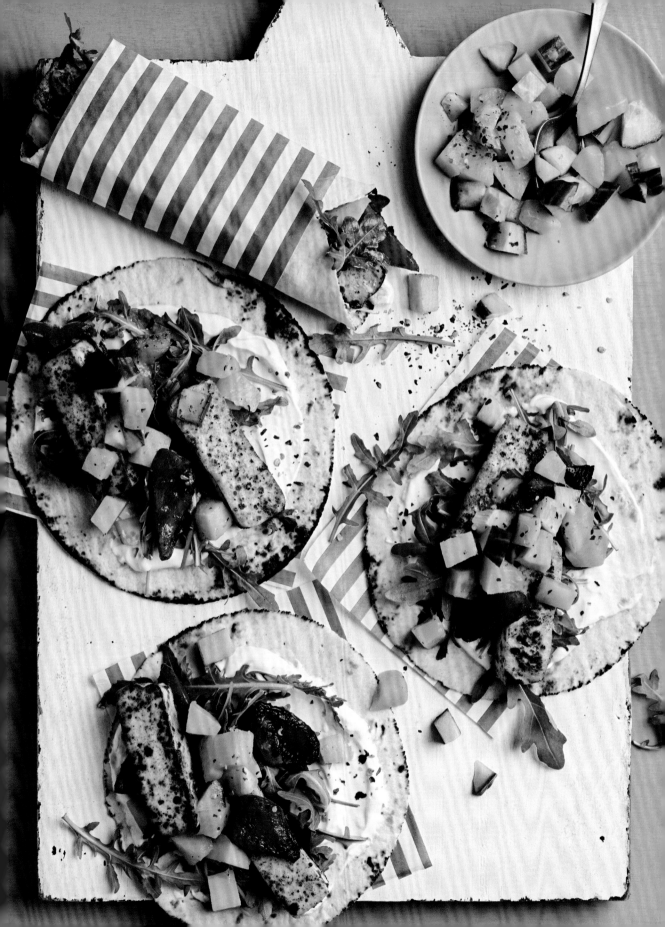

Halloumi + Sweet Pepper Gyros

Diversity points: 5 / Fibre: 4.3g

350g (12oz) full-fat live Greek yoghurt
3 large garlic cloves, grated or 2 heaped tsp garlic paste
15cm (6in) long piece of cucumber, sliced into half-moons
2 x 225g (8oz) blocks of halloumi cheese
200g (7oz) jarred peppers
2 tsp extra-virgin olive oil
1 tsp chilli flakes
4 round flatbreads
12 cos lettuce leaves, roughly torn
½ red onion, thinly sliced
Large handful of parsley leaves
Few mint leaves (optional)
Salt, to taste

+ Bonus Diversity Points

Add tomatoes and grated carrots to the wraps to boost the salad content.

The great thing about a block of halloumi is that it sits rather patiently at the back of the fridge ready for use when you need it most. Its long shelf life makes it an essential item in my fridge and here its dense saltiness contrasts with sweet roasted peppers and crunchy, garlicy cucumbers to make this the ultimate wrap of dreams.

1. Combine the Greek yoghurt and garlic in a bowl and then add the sliced cucumber, stir gently to combine and season with a little salt.

2. Pat the halloumi blocks dry with kitchen paper, then cut into slices about 1cm (½in) thick. Place a non-stick frying pan over a medium-high heat, add the halloumi slices and cook for 2 minutes on each side until the halloumi is golden brown all over.

3. While the halloumi is cooking roughly chop or tear the roasted peppers into strips and drizzle with olive oil and chilli flakes. Heat the flatbreads in the microwave or in another frying pan on the hob.

4. To assemble the gyros, spread the cucumber yoghurt over the base of each flatbread and add a handful of lettuce and some slices of onion. Top with the halloumi cheese and roasted peppers along with a handful of parsley and a few mint leaves (if using). Pack tightly into a roll and enjoy immediately.

Time Saving Hack
Instead of spending time chopping everything finely, just tear the lettuce leaves and herbs. The fine chopping makes near enough no difference to the final result.

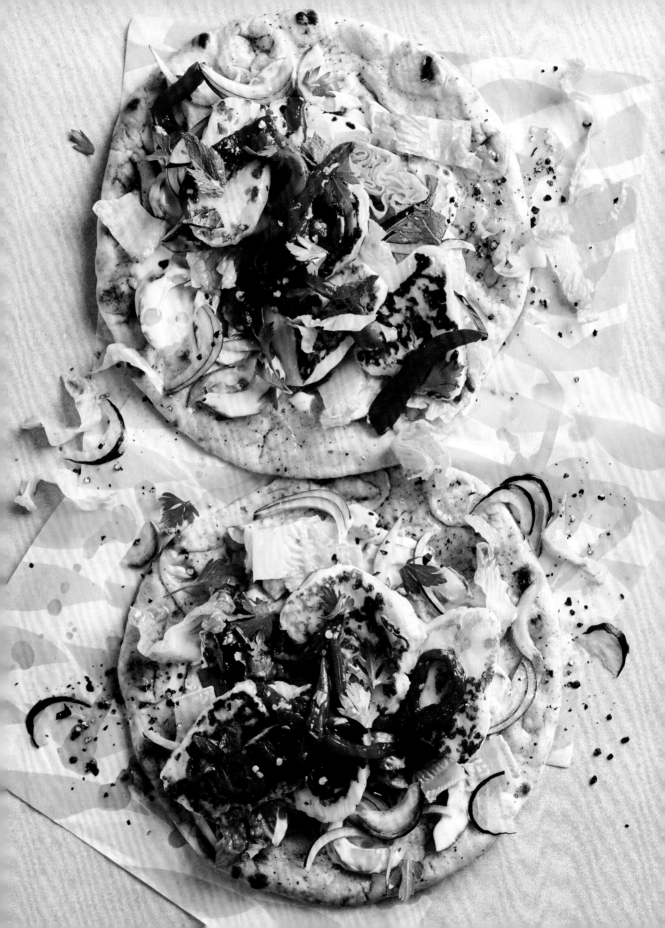

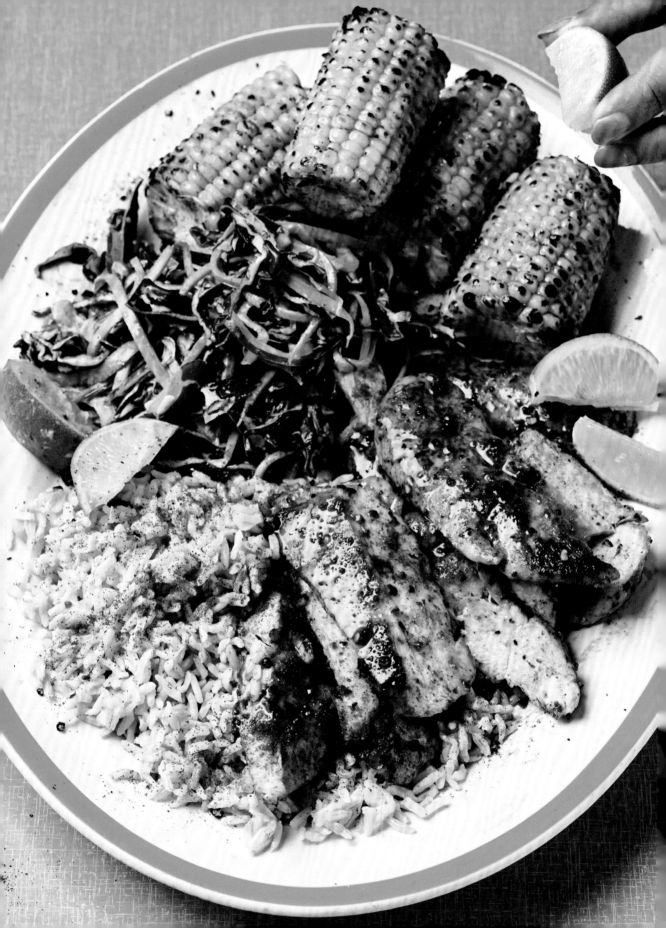

Peri Peri Chicken with All the Sides

Diversity points: 4 / Fibre: Xg

4 x 100–125g (3½–4oz) chicken breasts, about 1cm (½in) thick

1–2 tbsp peri peri rub

1 tbsp olive oil

Few flatbreads or leftover rice/grains/potatoes, to serve

FOR THE SWEETCORN

4 frozen corn cobs

1 tbsp extra-virgin olive oil

Salt, to taste

FOR THE SLAW

¼ red cabbage, finely shredded

1 large carrot, grated or julienned

½ red onion, thinly sliced

1 tsp peri peri rub

Juice of 1 lime

1–2 tbsp full-fat Greek yoghurt

Salt, to taste

+ Bonus Diversity Points

Serve alongside a grain salad dressed with pumpkin seeds, almonds and peas.

Time Saving Hack

Food processor slicing and grating attachments are a huge time-saver. Alternatively, you can buy pre-cut salad bags of coleslaw vegetables that you can then dress at home yourself.

Craving a peri peri chicken takeaway? Have I got a recipe for you! Minutes to get to the table and guaranteed satisfaction from everyone at the table, young and old. In the past I have made my own peri peri seasoning but the rubs available these days are of such high quality that I hardly need to spend time making my own. I would recommend a spice rub over a marinade from a bottle as there is a much higher chance of the marinades containing unwanted additives, making them ultra-processed.

1. Place the chicken breasts in a shallow bowl and dust the liberally with the peri peri rub. Drizzle over the olive oil and use your hands to rub the rub and oil all over the chicken.

2. Place a non-stick frying pan over a medium-high heat; when hot, add the chicken breasts and fry for 2–3 minutes on each side, or until the chicken is cooked through and the edges are golden and charred. (If you have an air fryer, you can roast the chicken in the air fryer at 200°C for 6–8 minutes.)

3. While the chicken is cooking place the frozen corn cobs in a microwave-safe bowl, splash with a little water and cook from frozen for about 8 minutes, or until tender. Drizzle the olive oil over the sweetcorn and season with salt to taste. If you have time, you can hold the corn with tongs near the flame of the hob and char slightly.

4. To make the slaw, put the sliced/shredded vegetables into a bowl and season with peri peri rub, salt and lime juice. Mix in the Greek yoghurt and stir well.

5. Serve the peri peri chicken with the all the sides.

Hot + Sour Aubergines with Cashews

Diversity points: 7 / Fibre: 6.5g

2 large aubergines, cut into 2.5cm (1in) chunks

4 generous tbsp vegetable oil

6 tbsp sriracha sauce

4 tbsp dark soy sauce

2 tbsp rice wine vinegar

1 tbsp maple syrup

1 heaped tsp garlic paste

1 heaped tsp ginger paste

1 heaped tbsp cornflour

250ml (9fl oz/1 cup) kettle-hot water

2 x 250g (9oz) pouches of pre-cooked jasmine/wild/brown rice

1 red pepper, cut into large chunks

1 yellow pepper, cut into large chunks

120g (4oz) roasted cashews

+ Bonus Diversity Points

Add spring onions or diced red onions to the aubergines and peppers and peas to the rice.

Time Saving Hack

To save precious time, you can prepare your hot and sour spice mixture in advance and have it ready to use in the fridge. If two of you are cooking together, one person can prepare the aubergines and the peppers and the other can prepare the sauce and cornflour slurry. This is a great way to really speed up the cooking.

Cold, dreary evenings just cry out for the hot and sour treatment. And though I have had hot and sour chicken or beef many times from a local takeaway, there really is no beating this version made with chunks of soft aubergine. Aubergines take a notoriously long time to cook so I've used my air fryer to cut the cooking time. If you don't have an air fryer, you can pan-fry the aubergines – just use plenty of oil and chop the aubergines into smaller pieces to save time.

1. Put the aubergine chunks into a bowl, drizzle with 3 tablespoons of the vegetable oil, season with salt and transfer to the air fryer. Roast at 200°C (400°F) for 14 minutes, opening the door of the air fryer and tossing the aubergines during cooking to ensure that they cook evenly.

2. Combine the sriracha, soy sauce, vinegar, maple syrup, ginger and garlic in a bowl. Mix the cornflour with the kettle-hot water to form a slurry and heat the rice in the microwave according to the instructions on the packet.

3. When the aubergines have finished roasting, place a wok over a high heat and add the remaining tablespoon of oil followed by the peppers. Stir-fry for about 2 minutes so that they acquire some colour and heat through. Toss in the aubergines from the air fryer followed by the prepared sauce. Stir well to combine everything.

4. Pour in the cornflour slurry and quickly bring to the boil, stirring constantly – the mixture will become thick and silky very quickly. Toss in the cashews and serve alongside the rice.

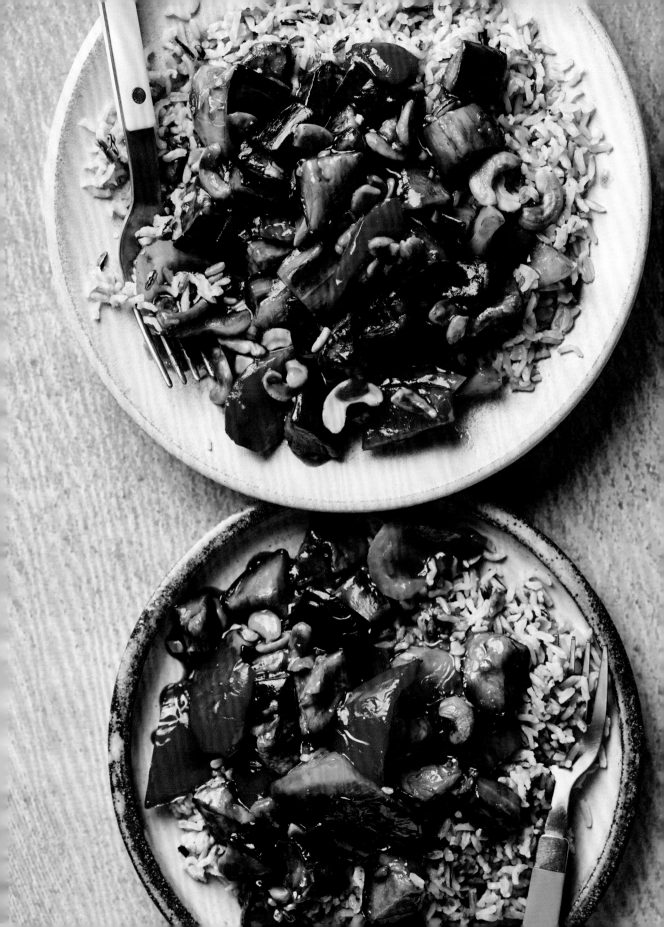

Jackfruit Pancakes

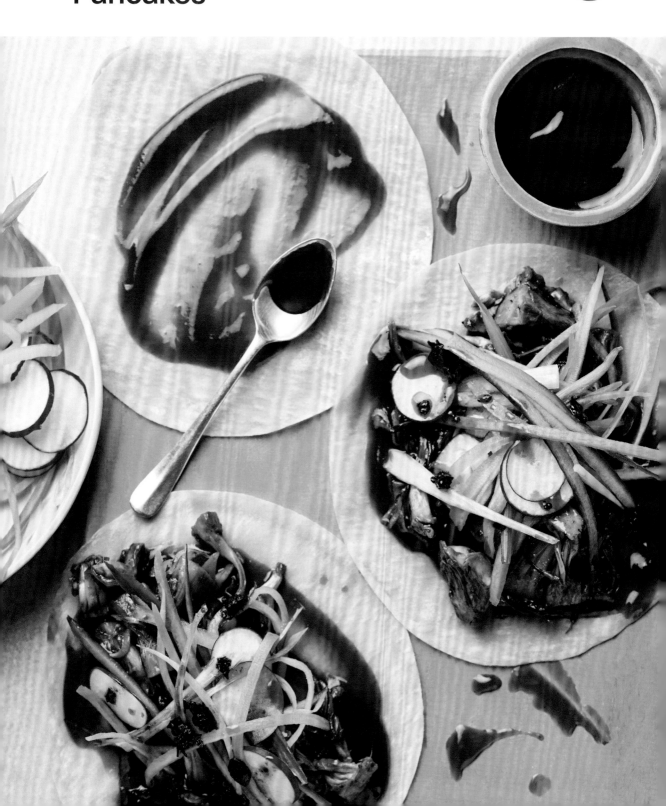

Diversity points: 8 / Fibre: 15g

24 frozen pancakes for crispy duck

2 x 400g (14oz) tins jackfruit

4 tbsp vegetable oil

2 tsp Chinese five-spice

1 tsp garlic paste

1 tsp ginger paste

8 tbsp hoisin sauce, plus extra to serve

15cm (6in) piece of cucumber

4 spring onions

1 carrot

8 radishes

Handful of coriander leaves, roughly torn (optional)

Crispy chillies in oil (optional)

+ Bonus Diversity Points
Add any vegetables you like to the pancakes, e.g. mushrooms instead of jackfruit, or beansprouts and water chestnuts to the salad.

Time Saving Hack
If you have an air fryer, you can prepare the jackfruit by adding the vegetable oil, five-spice, garlic and ginger to the jackfruit and air frying for 6–7 minutes at 200°C (400°F) before stirring through the hoisin sauce.

This is my version of the classic Peking duck dish, but far speedier and with many more added veggies! I buy the duck pancake wrappers from an oriental supermarket. They come in packets of 12 and are a useful little item to have stored away in the freezer. Tinned jackfruit is now available in most supermarkets and is a great alternative to meat in many dishes.

1. Start by draining the jackfruit and patting it dry with kitchen paper. Use your fingers to squash and tear the jackfruit into small pieces before patting dry again.

2. Place a frying pan over a medium-high heat and add the vegetable oil. When the oil is hot, but not yet smoking, add the jackfruit and fry for 4–5 minutes until it starts turning golden and slightly crispy at the edges.

3. Add the Chinese five-spice, garlic and ginger to the jackfruit and stir well to combine. After another minute or two add the hoisin sauce and stir well – the jackfruit should be a sticky consistency. It will only need a minute or two on the heat once the hoisin sauce has been added.

4. While the jackfruit is cooking cut the cucumber in half lengthways and remove the seeds, then slice the cucumber into long thin strips. Halve the spring onions lengthways and then cut into matchsticks. Peel the carrot and slice that into matchsticks as well. Thinly slice the radishes.

5. Place the pancakes in the microwave for 30–60 seconds until they have defrosted and are steaming and easy to separate (check the instructions on the packet). Keep the pancakes warm by wrapping in a tea towel until you are ready to eat them.

6. Put everything on the table so that everyone can assemble their own pancakes. Start by spreading extra hoisin sauce over the base of a pancake, then top with the jackfruit, cucumbers, spring onions, carrots and radishes. Finish with some coriander and some crisp chillies in oil, if you like. Roll into a pancake and enjoy.

Sunshine Carrot, Coriander + Halloumi Frittata

Light
Suppers

Diversity points: 6 / Fibre: 7.3g

3 generous tbsp olive oil
250g (9oz) carrots, grated
2 tsp cumin seeds
350g (12oz) halloumi, cut into small cubes
3 tbsp harissa paste
6 medium or 5 large eggs
Large handful of coriander leaves, roughly torn

TO SERVE

Rocket leaves dressed with a squeeze of lemon juice
A few slices of toasted sourdough

+ Bonus Diversity Points

Add leftover brassicas like cabbage, cauliflower or broccoli to you frittata, or even thinly sliced onions and leeks.

Time Saving Hack

By using harissa paste you decrease the time spent reaching for all the spices in the store cupboard. It is a very versatile spice mix that I would recommend to any and every cook.

The frittata is one of those dishes that can never lose its appeal. This is probably because it is open to endless interpretation, you can virtually add any of your favourite ingredients or leftover vegetables from the fridge to the egg base.
Here I use a pack of pre-grated carrots from my local supermarket. I don't expect you to buy your carrots grated, but it does save me a lot of time and energy.

1. Heat the olive oil in a large (30cm/12in) non-stick frying pan over a medium heat and add the grated carrot and cumin seeds. Fry for 3–4 minutes until the carrot starts to soften.

2. Increase the heat to high and add the halloumi to the pan. Stir well to combine, keeping the heat high so that the halloumi pieces gain a slightly golden colour and the carrots do not stew. Stir the harissa paste through the carrots and halloumi.

3. Beat the eggs in a bowl, add the coriander leaves and then pour the egg mixture over the carrot and halloumi. Reduce the heat to medium and cook through for 5 minutes, then carefully flip over and cook for a final 2 minutes. You're looking for a deep golden-brown colour on the surface of the frittata. If you find it hard to flip the frittata in the pan, turn it out on to a plate first and then gently slide it back into the pan. Alternatively, you can finish cooking the dish under a hot grill until the surface is bubbling and golden.

4. Serve the frittata hot, warm or at room temperature, with the rocket leaves and toasted sourdough on the side.

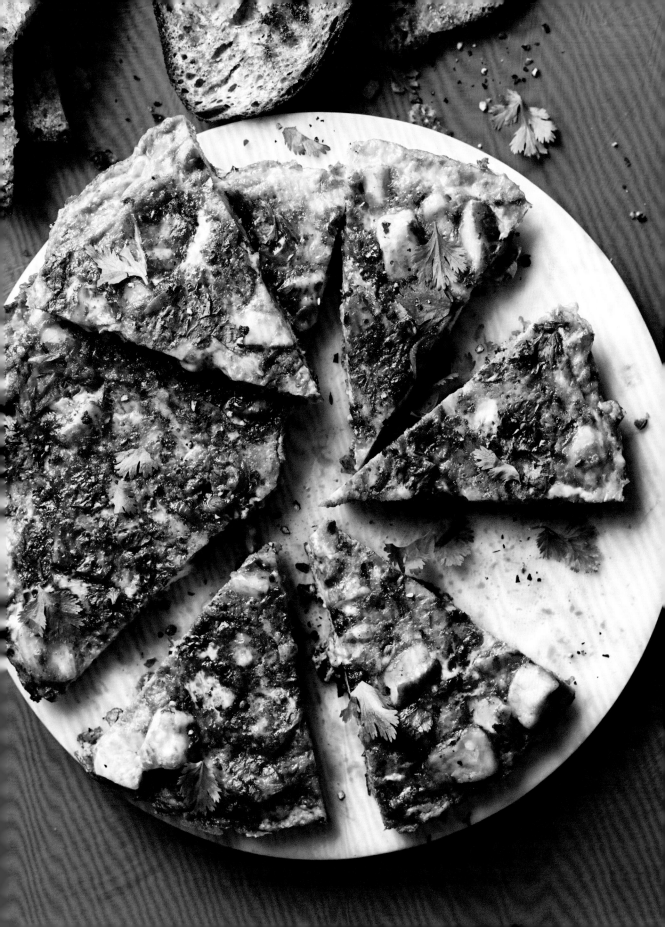

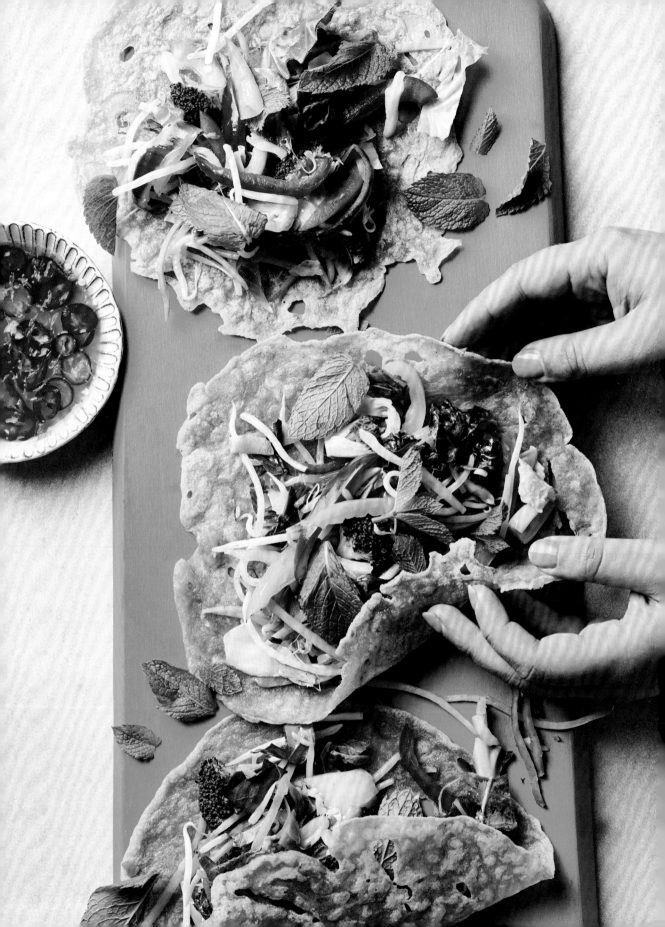

Vietnamese-Style Crispy Pancakes with Stir-Fry Veg

Light
Suppers

Diversity points: 7 / Fibre: 2.4g

FOR THE PANCAKES

75g (2¾oz) cornflour

200ml (7fl oz/generous ¾ cup) coconut milk

2–3 ice cubes

1 tsp ground turmeric

Vegetable oil, for frying

Salt, to taste

FOR THE FILLING

1 tbsp vegetable oil

320g (11oz) stir-fry vegetables

FOR THE DIPPING SAUCE

3 tbsp fish sauce

Juice of 2 limes

2 tsp sugar

6 tbsp water

1–2 chillies, finely chopped

+ Bonus Diversity Points

*Add soft herbs like roughly torn coriander and mint
leaves to your pancakes for an extra punch of flavour.*

Time Saving Hack

*You can prepare the batter (minus the ice cubes) in
advance and have it ready to go in the fridge.*

A mixed bag of stir-fry vegetables is highly underrated. To me it epitomises convenient, gut-friendly eating: all vegetables are cut and prepared for you and you'll find at least five different vegetables in each pack, contributing to diversity in your diet. Stir-fry veg also has a minimal cooking time, appealing to my indolent side. However, I can become bored of plain vegetable stir-fry, which is why this recipe for crispy pancakes with an umami-rich Vietnamese-style dipping sauce really hits the spot.

1. Put the cornflour, coconut milk, ice cubes, turmeric and a pinch of salt into a bowl or jug and stir well to combine.

2. Heat a large frying pan over a medium heat and brush with a little oil. Ladle a quarter of the mixture into the pan and spread it over the base to make a thin, crepe-like pancake about 20cm (8in) in diameter. When it looks like it has cooked through, after about 2 minutes, flip over and cook for another couple of minutes. The edges of the pancake should be quite crisp. Repeat the process to make four pancakes, adding more oil to the pan as needed.

3. While you are cooking the pancakes, heat the vegetable oil in a wok over a medium heat and add the stir-fry vegetables and a pinch of salt. Stir-fry for 2–3 minutes until the vegetables are just cooked through but still crisp.

4. Put the fish sauce, lime juice, sugar and water into a small bowl and stir well to combine before adding the chopped chilli.

5. To assemble the pancakes stuff them with the stir-fried vegetables and serve with the dipping sauce on the side.

Speedy Green Bean, Garlic + Tomato Stew

Light
Suppers

Diversity points: 4 / Fibre: 8.9g

3 tbsp extra-virgin olive oil

2 tsp garlic paste (or 3 garlic cloves, grated)

500g (1lb 2oz) green beans

250g (9oz) good-quality passata

Few sprigs of thyme, leaves picked

175ml (6fl oz/¾ cup) kettle-hot water

250g (9oz) cherry tomatoes

1 tsp honey or sugar (optional)

Salt and pepper, to taste

TO SERVE

Sourdough baguette

Large handful of watercress, dressed with a squeeze of lemon juice

Goats' cheese (optional)

+ Bonus Diversity Points

Add mangetout and peas to your bean stew and serve with a salad of finely sliced fennel and red onions with lemon juice and capers over the top, and a touch of salt and olive oil.

How can something so simple taste so utterly delicious? This recipe has year-long appeal, equally comforting in spring, summer, autumn and winter. A good-quality passata (with minimal added ingredients) is essential for a delicious result. You can serve the dish with grains like bulgur wheat or spelt if you prefer this to bread.

1. Place a wide-mouthed saucepan or cast-iron casserole dish over a medium heat and add 2 tablespoons of the olive oil. Add the garlic and once it starts to turn golden add the green beans and fry for 2–3 minutes.

2. Add the passata, thyme leaves and hot water and season with salt and pepper. Simmer for 7–8 minutes until the green beans soften and turn a darker green colour.

3. Add the cherry tomatoes to the pan for the last 2 minutes of cooking and allow them to swell and blister. Taste the green beans – if they are too acidic add a teaspoon of honey or sugar to balance out the flavour.

4. Drizzle the remaining tablespoon of extra-virgin olive oil over the stew, then serve with sliced sourdough, watercress and goats' cheese, if liked.

Time Saving Hack
Chopping your green beans and using a wide-mouthed saucepan will speed up the cooking time significantly.

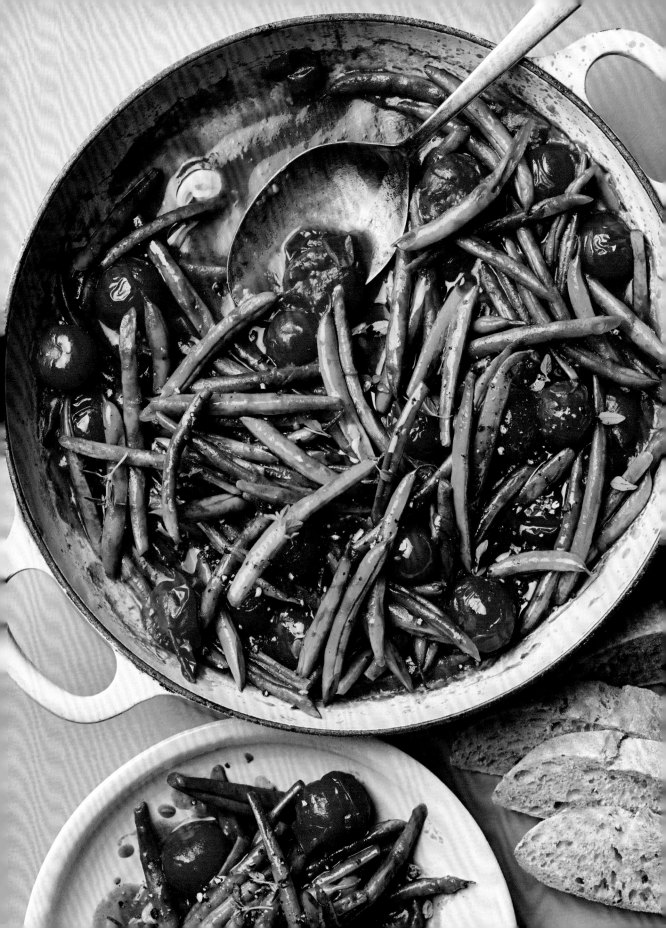

Gut-Loving Pesto with Chicken + Greens

Diversity points: 7 / Fibre: 7.7g

1 tbsp vegetable oil

4 x 125–150g (4–5oz) chicken breast steaks, 1–1.5cm (½in) thick

200g (7oz) frozen peas

100g (3½oz) green beans

Crusty bread or pre-cooked grains (from a pouch), to serve

FOR THE PESTO

75g (2¾oz) spinach leaves

30g (1oz) basil leaves

1 tbsp garlic paste

50g (2oz) toasted hazelnuts

75g (2¾oz) Parmesan cheese (or vegetarian hard cheese)

100ml (3½fl oz/scant ½ cup) extra-virgin olive oil

+ Bonus Diversity Points
Add a handful of cherry tomatoes to the pan at the last minute. Serve with a mixed leaf salad dressed with lemon juice.

Time Saving Hack
Making more pesto than you need will save you time another day. Try adding to cooked pasta, cherry tomatoes and rocket leaves for a lovely pasta salad dish, ideal for lunch. Or thinly slice 1 leek and 1 courgette and lightly fry in olive oil before adding a tin of drained white beans, a packet of shop-bought ravioli and 200ml (7fl oz/generous ¾ cup) of water to cook the ravioli through. Spoon over the leftover pesto and serve.

Pesto, but given the gut-health treatment. This is one of the dishes that has the potential to become a real family favourite. I deliberately make more pesto than is needed here as leftover pesto can be used in so many fun ways – I have given a few ideas below. To keep the short cooking time, make sure the chicken breast steaks are no more than 1–1.5cm (½in) thick.

1. Put the spinach, basil, garlic, hazelnuts and Parmesan into a food processor and blitz until well combined. Pour in the extra-virgin olive oil and blitz for a few more seconds to create the pesto.

2. Place a wide, flat non-stick frying pan over a high heat and drizzle in the vegetable oil. Add the chicken to the hot pan and fry for 3–4 minutes until the underside turns golden. Turn the chicken breasts over and spoon a heaped tablespoon of the pesto on top of each one. Add about 5 tablespoons of kettle-hot water to the pan and baste the chicken with the water to form a thick, vivid green sauce that coats the chicken. The chicken will only need a further minute or two to cook through.

3. Put the peas and green beans into a microwave-safe bowl and microwave on high for 5 minutes, or until cooked through.

4. Serve the chicken and greens with crusty bread or grains of your choice.

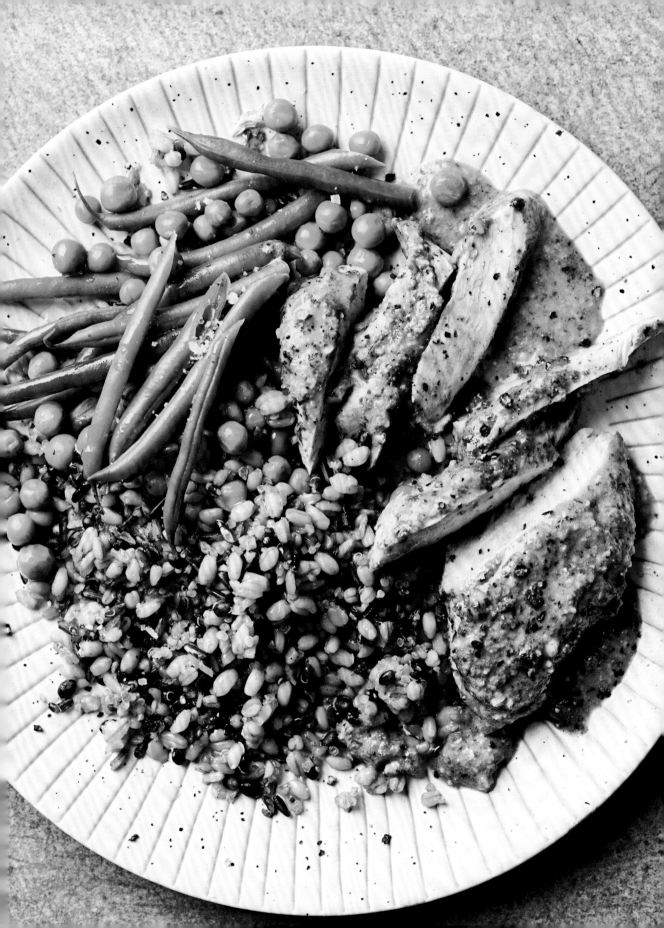

Summery Tomato Curry with Cucumber Raita + Chapatti

Diversity points: 8 / Fibre: 5.9g

I make this recipe when everyone's in the mood for curry but there's not much in the fridge apart from tomatoes and slightly floppy cucumbers. And goodness, do they transform for the better. Though I nearly always advocate the use of ginger paste from a jar for ease, fresh ginger really does make a difference in this recipe.

4 tbsp olive oil

2 small white onions, diced

4 garlic cloves, thinly sliced

2 x thumb-sized pieces of ginger, peeled and julienned

2 green chillies, chopped

1 tsp red chilli powder

1 tsp ground coriander

1 tsp cumin seeds

1 tsp mustard seeds

800g (1lb 12oz) cherry tomatoes

4–6 frozen wholewheat chapattis

250g (9oz) full-fat live Greek yoghurt

15cm (6in) piece of cucumber

Few sprigs of coriander and/or mint leaves

Salt, to taste

+ Bonus Diversity Points
Add cooked diced potatoes, black chickpeas or black-eyed peas to the tomatoes. For those looking to increase their protein intake, a fried egg makes a worthy addition.

Time Saving Hack
I always have frozen chapattis in my freezer. They are made of just two ingredients - whole wheat flour and water - and cook in minutes from frozen in a non-stick frying pan. You can of course use pitta bread, naan or other flatbreads of your choice.

1. Heat the olive oil in a non-stick frying pan over a medium-high heat and add the olive oil. When the oil is hot but not yet smoking add the onions, garlic and ginger.

2. When the onions start to brown and soften slightly (this takes around 4-5 minutes) add the green chillies, chilli powder, ground coriander and cumin and mustard seeds. Stir well to prevent the spices catching. Add two-thirds of the cherry tomatoes; slice the remaining third and then add these to the pan too. Season with salt to taste. Cook the tomatoes through for just 2–3 minutes so that they warm through and start to blister but do not break down completely.

3. Meanwhile, warm the chapattis according to the packet instructions. Tip the Greek yoghurt into a bowl and grate in the cucumber. Add any leftover herbs like coriander or mint to the raita and season with salt to taste.

4. Serve the tomato curry straight from the pan with the chapattis and cucumber raita on the side.

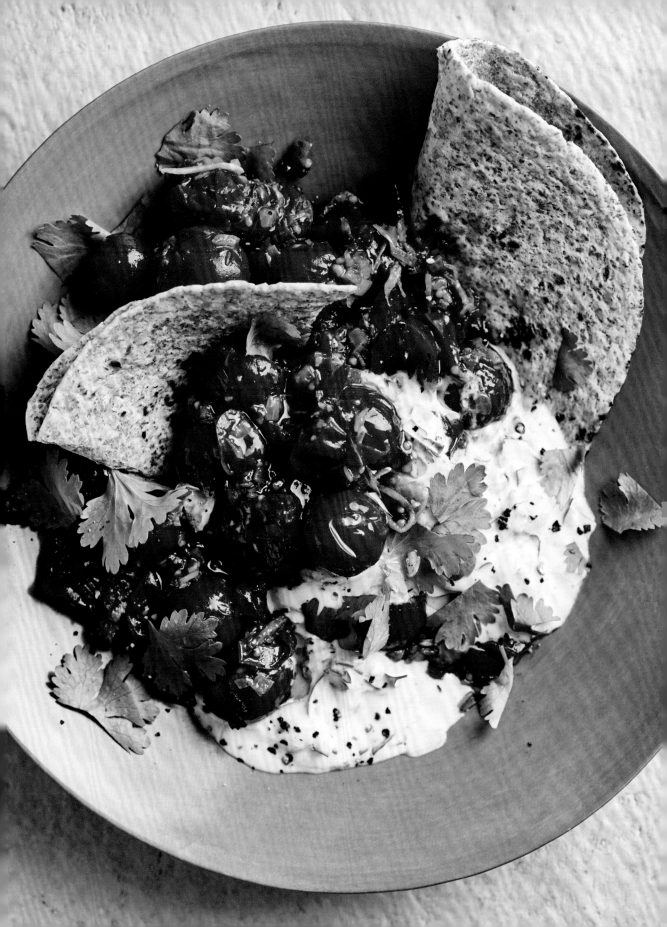

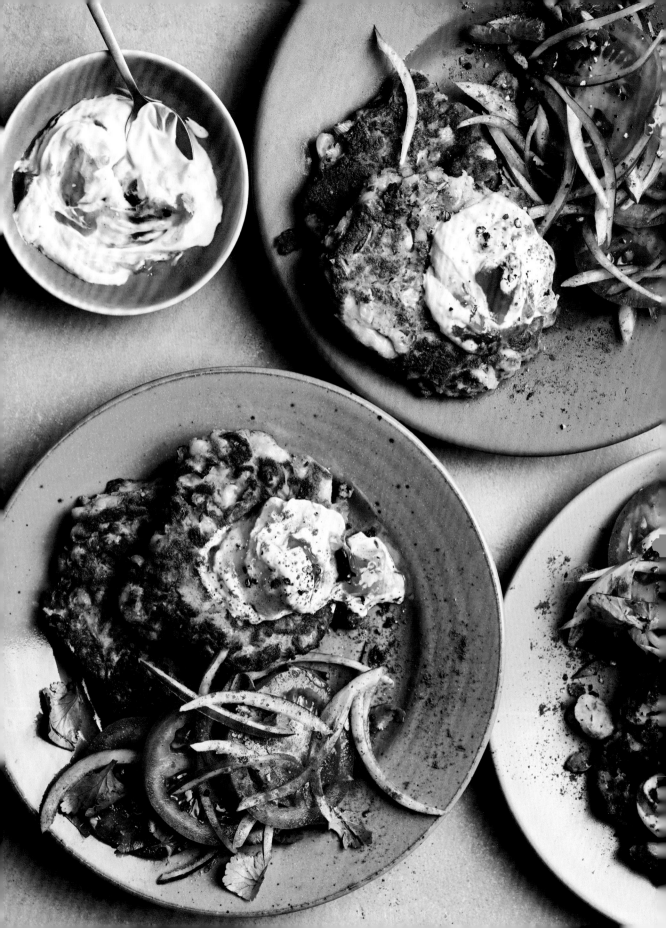

Spiced Cannellini Bean Fritters

Light
Suppers

Diversity points: 6 / Fibre: 6.7g

2 x 400g (14oz) tins cannellini beans, drained and rinsed

2 tbsp jalfrezi paste

½ tsp ground turmeric

½ tsp cumin seeds

Handful of coriander leaves, roughly chopped

1 egg

1 spring onion, thinly sliced

2 tbsp cornflour or plain flour

Vegetable oil, for frying

Salt, to taste

TO SERVE

150g (5oz) full-fat live Greek yoghurt

6 tsp mango chutney

2 ripe tomatoes, thickly sliced

½ red onion, thinly sliced

½ tsp chilli powder (*optional*)

Handful coriander leaves, roughly torn

+ Bonus Diversity Points

Instead of using just cannellini beans, use half kidney beans and half cannellini beans. Leftover broccoli and cauliflower would also work well in this recipe.

Time Saving Hack

Using a paste means you won't have to rummage for individual spices – korma, tandoori or vindaloo pastes work well. Try and avoid preservatives, artificial colours and emulsifiers and look for ones that are just spices in oil.

Dense, spicy, warm and moreish. What more could one ask for from a bean fritter? On days where I want a light supper, I serve these with a simple salad and maybe a few warmed grains. But, if you're in the mood for something more substantial, the fritters also make for a wonderful burger filling with lots of salad and lashings of mango chutney.

1. Use a kitchen towel to pat the drained beans dry before transferring them to a large bowl. Add the jalfrezi paste, turmeric, cumin seeds, coriander leaves, egg and spring onion and use a fork to mix everything together, pressing down on the beans to mash them slightly. Add the cornflour to the mixture and stir again. Season with salt to taste.

2. Place a non-stick frying pan over a medium heat and drizzle in a teaspoon or two of vegetable oil. Spoon the bean mixture into the pan to form fritters that are 8–10cm (3–4in) wide and 2cm (¾in) thick. Fry for 2 minutes on each side, turning them carefully to ensure that they don't fall apart, although the egg should help them hold together.

3. Place the yoghurt in a small bowl, season with a pinch of salt and spoon over the mango chutney. Use the back of a spoon to marble the mango chutney into the yoghurt. Combine the sliced tomatoes, onion and coriander and sprinkle with a pinch of salt and a little chilli powder (if using).

4. Serve the fritters with the tomato and onion salad on the side and the mango chutney yoghurt for dipping.

Steamed Fish with Greens

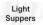

Light Suppers

Diversity points: 4 / Fibre: 3.9g

4 x 200g (7oz) cod fillets, about 3cm (1¼in) thick

2 large thumb-sized pieces of ginger, peeled and julienned

2 tbsp rice wine vinegar

6 tbsp soy sauce

4 tbsp water

2 tsp maple syrup or honey

2 pak choi, quartered lengthways

300g (10oz) sugar snap peas

2 spring onions, shredded lengthways

3 tbsp vegetable oil

2 x 250g (9oz) pouches of jasmine rice, to serve

TO GARNISH (OPTIONAL)

2 tsp toasted sesame oil

2 tsp chilli oil

Handful of roughly torn coriander

+ Bonus Diversity Points
Consider adding broccoli or even mushrooms to the fish while it's steaming.

Time Saving Hack
If you are using frozen fish (it can be much more economical) then make sure you defrost it fully in the fridge before using.

A light and sophisticated dinner dish. Though subtle, it packs a punch in flavour with an elegant umami tone. You can use any fish of your choice including salmon, haddock or tilapia. I have used skinless cod fillets for ease.

1. Prepare your steaming apparatus – I usually place a heatproof dish on a stand inside a large pan that has a tight-fitting lid and pour kettle-hot water into the base of the pan, making sure it won't touch the heatproof dish.

2. Place the fish fillets into the heatproof dish and scatter over the ginger strips. Combine the vinegar, soy sauce, water and maple syrup in a small bowl and pour this over the fish. Place the dish in the steamer and place the steamer over a medium-high heat.

3. When the fish has been steaming for 3 minutes, add the pak choi quarters and scatter the sugar snap peas into the dish, around the fish fillets. Steam for a further 4 minutes.

4. While your fish and veg is steaming, gently heat the vegetable oil in a small saucepan. Heat the jasmine rice in a microwave, according to the packet instructions.

5. Carefully remove the heatproof dish from the steamer. Scatter the spring onions over the fish and then pour over the hot oil – it will sizzle a little. Although this step isn't essential, I'm told it's authentic and traditional. Serve with the jasmine rice. If you like, drizzle with sesame oil and chilli oil and scatter over some roughly torn coriander.

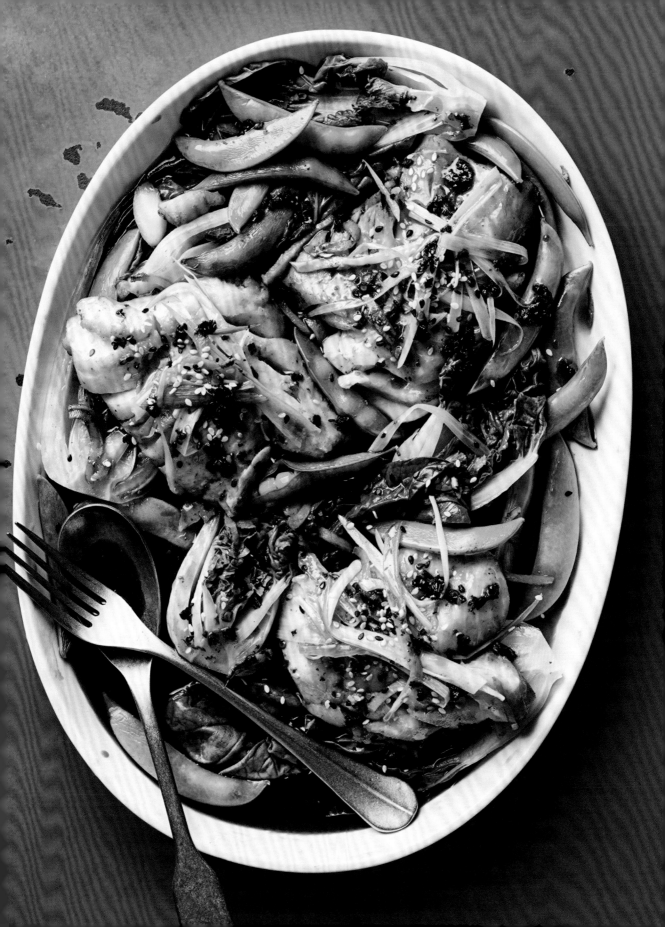

Chilli Peanut
Silken Tofu
with Rice

Diversity points: 5 / Fibre: 3.7g

300g (10oz) block of silken tofu

2 tbsp soy sauce

1 tsp garlic paste

1 tbsp crunchy peanut butter

1 tsp chilli oil

1 spring onion, thinly sliced

10cm (4in) piece of cucumber, sliced into long ribbons

1 tbsp sesame seeds (optional)

250g (9oz) pouch of cooked jasmine rice

+ Bonus Diversity Points
Steam some mangetout, green beans or pak choi to enjoy alongside the tofu and rice.

Cartons of silken tofu can be bought in most supermarkets these days. Silken tofu doesn't need to be refrigerated and can sit ready for use in your store cupboard. It has a really smooth texture and is a great protein-rich alternative to eggs.

1. Carefully open the silken tofu, sliding it out of the carton, and cut into 2.5cm slices.

2. To make the sauce, combine the soy sauce, garlic and peanut butter in a bowl and add 3–3 tablespoons of kettle-hot water. Stir together to make a runny sauce.

3. Drizzle the sauce over the tofu and top with chilli oil, sliced spring onion, cucumber strips and sesame seeds (if using). Serve with jasmine rice, heated through in the microwave.

 Time Saving Hack
Make the peanut and soy sauce ahead of time and have it in your fridge ready to go. It also makes a wonderful dipping sauce for crudités.

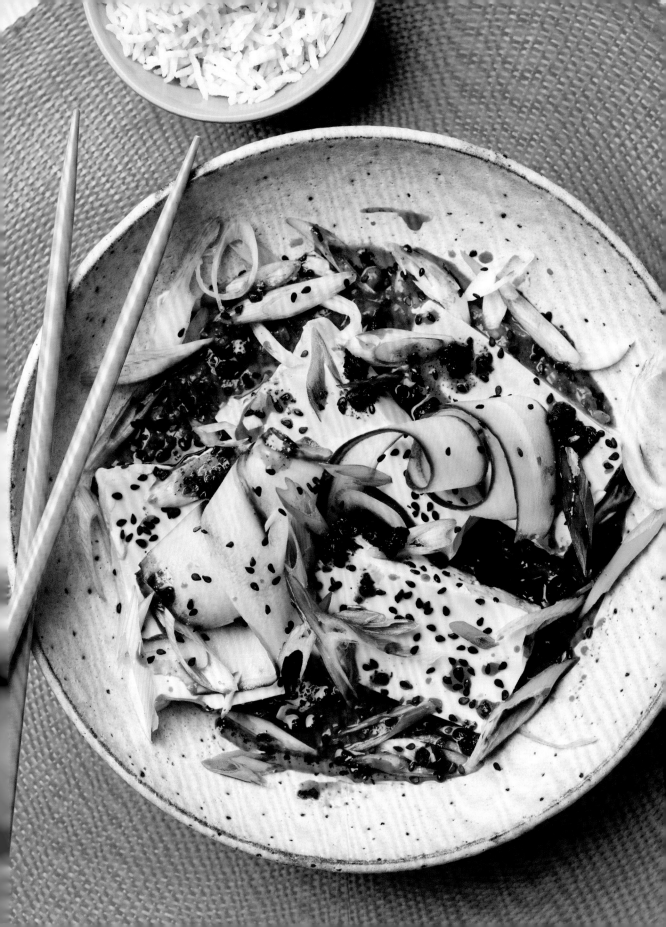

Spinach, Kefir + Walnut Soup with Crusty Sourdough

Diversity points: 4 / Fibre: 13g

100g (3½oz) walnuts
1 garlic clove
2 tbsp vegetable oil
150ml (5fl oz/⅔ cup) kettle-hot water
400g (14oz) frozen chopped spinach, defrosted
2 x 400g (14oz) tins green lentils, drained and rinsed
800g (1lb 12oz) kefir yoghurt
Pinch of chilli flakes
Salt, to taste

+ Bonus Diversity Points
Serve your soup alongside some radishes. Experiment with using cooked beetroot instead of spinach. Add cooked grains like pearl barley or spelt to the soup.

The earthy walnut base of this soup pairs perfectly with the dense minerally flavour of spinach and lactic tang of kefir. I really think this could be one of the easiest soups of all time to make and – even better – it is full of probiotic kefir goodness.

1. Start by blitzing the walnuts and garlic clove in a spice grinder or food processor until a sandy consistency.

2. Heat the vegetable oil in a saucepan over a medium heat, add the walnuts and cook, stirring, for about 2 minutes, or until they start releasing a nutty aroma: make sure the nuts don't catch.

3. Add the hot water to the walnuts along with the spinach and lentils and stir thoroughly. Simmer for another minute or two until the lentils have warmed through.

4. Turn the heat down really low and add the kefir, stirring well to combine. Season with the chilli flakes and salt. When the soup has warmed through but is not quite boiling yet take it off the heat and pour it into serving bowls.

 Time Saving Hack
Blitz the walnuts and garlic in advance and have it ready for use. Frozen spinach is a real hero ingredient: because it comes ready chopped it will save you time but it's also very inexpensive while remaining nutritious. It will defrost in a microwave in about 1–1½ minutes.

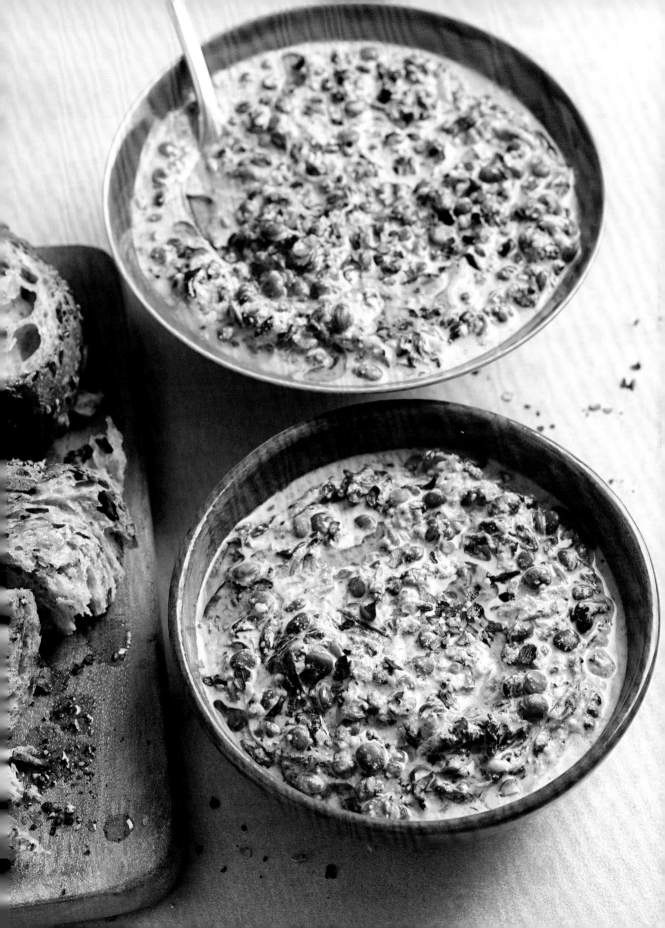

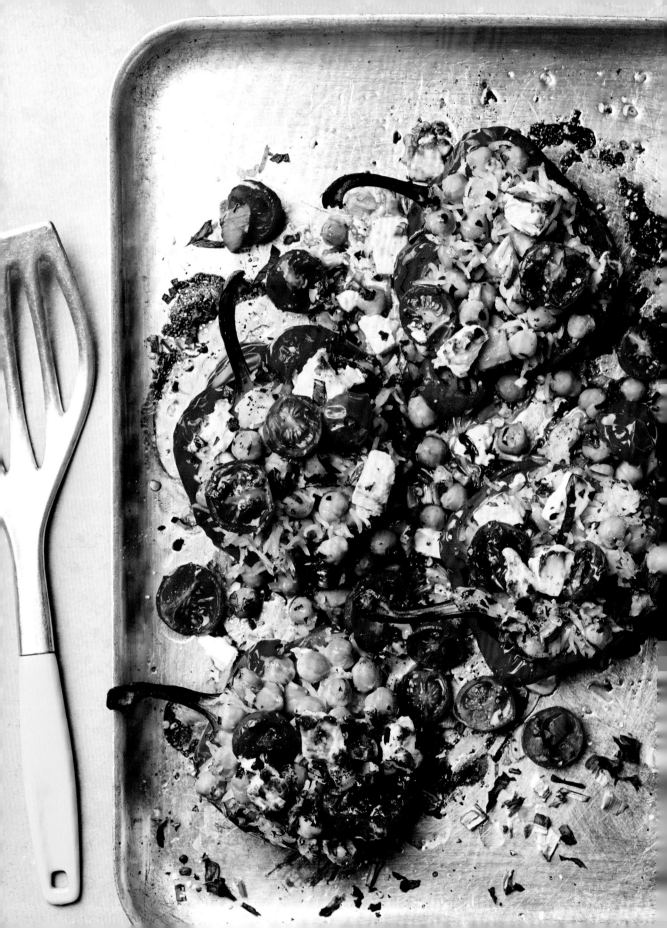

Greek Salad
Stuffed Peppers

Diversity points: 7 / Fibre: 14g

2 red peppers
2 tbsp extra-virgin olive oil, plus extra for drizzling
100g (3½oz) leftover cooked rice or other grain
½ x 400g (14oz) tin chickpeas, drained and rinsed
1 tsp garlic paste
1 tsp dried oregano
½ tsp red chilli flakes
½ red onion, diced
Handful of parsley, chopped
150g (5oz) cherry tomatoes, halved
100g (3½oz) feta cheese
Salt, to taste

+ Bonus Diversity Points
Serve with a salad of rocket leaves and toasted pine nuts or seeds.

Time Saving Hack
I use roasted peppers a lot in my dishes and they are great to prep ahead. If you ever have a free afternoon and lots of peppers to hand, simply drizzle them in olive oil and roast them, either in the air fryer or oven. Once cool, you can then place them a bowl, cover the peppers with clingfilm and slip off the skins. Transfer these peppers to a jar, top with olive oil and store in the fridge – they will keep well for about a fortnight.

This recipe happened when Greek salad met a few leftover grains and ended up being stuffed into a sweet pepper. This combination of Mediterranean flavours hits the spot every time and makes a perfect dish for alfresco dining (if the British weather allows). I use an air fryer to save time but you can also use a conventional oven. If you are doubling up the quantities to serve four, you will need a larger air fryer; alternatively just use the oven.

1. Halve the peppers lengthways, remove the seeds and core and rub them with about a tablespoon of the olive oil. Transfer to the air fryer and roast for 5 minutes at 200°C (400°F). (Alternatively, roast for 10 minutes in a conventional oven preheated to the same temperature.)

2. While the peppers are roasting, combine the cooked rice, chickpeas, garlic, oregano, chilli flakes and the remaining olive oil and season with salt to taste.

3. Remove the tray holding the peppers from the air fryer and carefully spoon this rice mixture into the peppers. Stud the surface of the stuffed peppers with the diced red onion, parsley and tomatoes, then crumble over the feta and drizzle with a little extra olive oil. Return to the air fryer for 6–8 minutes at 200°C (400°F) for a perfect stuffed pepper (or 10 minutes in a conventional oven).

Roast Cabbage with Sweet + Sour Peppers + Sultanas

Diversity points: 8 / Fibre: 18g

⅔ white cabbage (about 700g/1lb 9oz)

3 tbsp extra-virgin olive oil

250g (9oz) jarred peppers, roughly sliced

75g (2¾oz/½ cup) sultanas

3 tbsp apple cider vinegar

1 tsp chilli flakes

1 heaped tsp honey

1 x 400g (14oz) tin green/brown lentils, drained and rinsed

250g (9oz) pouch of pre-cooked mixed grains

60g (2½oz/⅓ cup) almonds, roughly chopped

75g (2¾oz) feta cheese, crumbled

25g (1oz) parsley, roughly chopped

Salt and pepper, to taste

+ Bonus Diversity Points

Add more nuts and seeds like hazelnuts, pine nuts and sunflower seeds for an extra crunchy topping. Use a combination of grains and tinned lentils or chickpeas to optimise the protein content of your dish.

Time Saving Hack

I use the air fryer to save time, but you can also cook the cabbage in a large non-stick frying pan placed over a high heat. Alternatively, try chopping the cabbage more finely and sautéing in a wok.

I'm not sure when it became fashionable to roast cabbage, but I am very glad it did. I use sweet-and-sour peppers and sultanas to make an express 'agrodolce' inspired dressing for the cabbage. You can make the dish more substantial by serving with any grains and lentils you have to hand.

1. Cut the cabbage into wedges that are no thicker than 2.5cm (1in), trying to keep the stalk on where you can. Splash a bit of water on to the cabbage - this will create steam and cook it through more evenly. Drizzle with the extra-virgin olive oil and season with salt and pepper, then transfer to the air fryer. Roast the cabbage for 10–12 minutes at 180°C (350°F), checking the progress by opening the air fryer door halfway through cooking and turning the cabbage over so all surfaces are exposed to the heat.

2. Meanwhile, put the roasted peppers into a small saucepan along with the sultanas, apple cider vinegar, chilli flakes and honey. Place over a low heat until it is thick and sticky, this takes just a minute or two.

3. Put the drained lentils in a microwave-safe bowl along with the mixed grains and heat in the microwave for 2–3 minutes until piping hot.

4. Spread the warmed lentils and grains over the base of a platter and top with the roasted cabbage wedges, then spoon over the sweet-and-sour peppers and sultanas. For a final flourish, scatter over the almonds, feta and parsley.

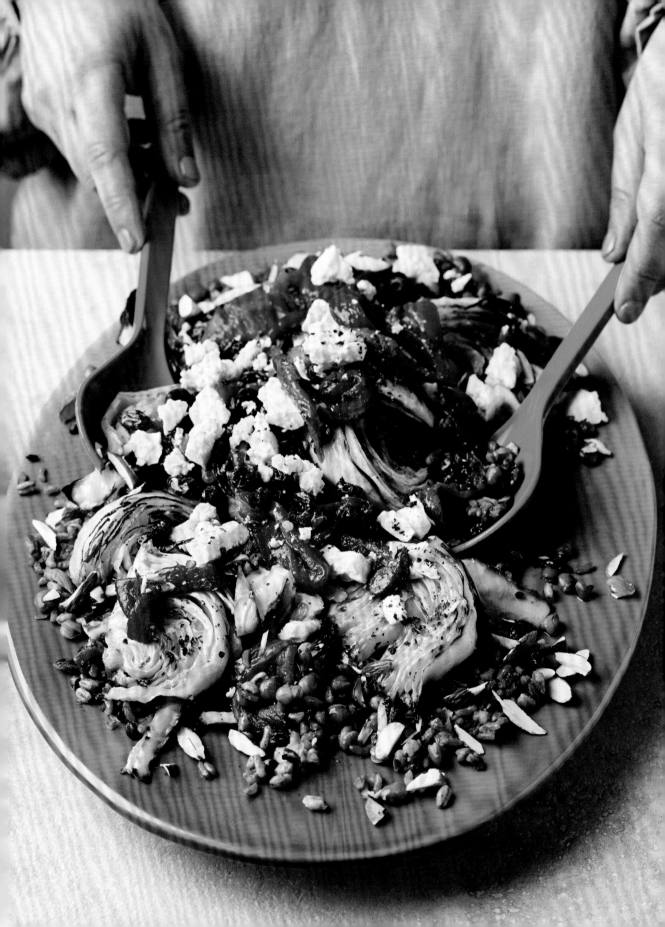

Crispy Seedy Fried Chicken with Gochujang Honey Sauce + Slaw

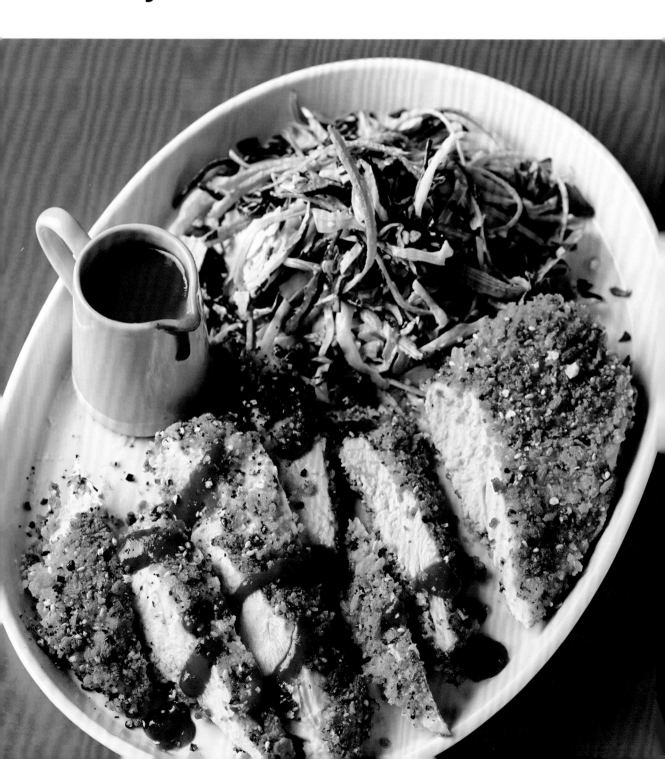

Diversity points: 7 / Fibre: 7.9g

4 x 150g (5oz) chicken breasts, no thicker than 1cm (½in)

2 eggs

2 heaped tbsp cornflour

200g (7oz/1½ cups) dried breadcrumbs

2 heaped tbsp sesame seeds (black, white or a combination)

2 tbsp chia seeds

2 tbsp flaxseeds

6 tbsp veg oil

275g (9¾oz) shop-bought crunchy coleslaw mix (discard any dressing)

Juice of 1 large lime

2 tsp sesame oil

4 tbsp gochujang paste

2 tsp honey

Salt, to taste

+ Bonus Diversity Points
You can serve with an array of steamed vegetables of your choice. Broccoli, green beans and pak choi would make a good side too.

Time Saving Hack
Instead of doing a classic 'pane' where you have to coat chicken in flour, then egg, then breadcrumbs, I just make a sticky paste with the eggs and cornflour and dunk the coated chicken straight into the crumbs. This creates less washing up and is much quicker too.

This is my version of a gut-healthy chicken schnitzel, crunchy, seedy and satisfying. It is drizzled with a sweet, sticky, spicy sauce of dreams made from a Korean spice paste called Gochujang. Well worth investing in a good Gochujang paste as its completely addictive and you will find yourself turning to it time and time again!

1. Start by putting the chicken into a bowl and seasoning generously with salt. Crack the eggs into the bowl and then add the cornflour. Give the mixture a really good stir so that the chicken is coated with a sticky eggy, cornflour paste.

2. Combine the breadcrumbs, sesame seeds, chia seeds and flaxseeds on a separate tray and stir well to combine.

3. Place a large non-stick frying pan over a medium heat and add the oil to the pan. Carefully drop the chicken into the breadcrumb/seed mixture and turn to ensure that all of the chicken is coated in the crumbs. Transfer the breadcrumbed chicken to the frying pan and fry for about 4 minutes on each side, or until they are a deep golden colour and completely cooked through.

4. While the chicken is cooking, prepare the coleslaw by placing the mixed coleslaw vegetables in a bowl with the lime juice, sesame oil and salt to taste. Give the vegetables a good scrunch with your hands to help get the flavours all the way through the veg.

5. Put the gochujang paste, honey and 175ml (6fl oz/¾ cup) water into a small saucepan and bring it to the boil, then simmer until it is sticky and thick – this only takes a minute or two.

6. Serve the chicken with the coleslaw and gochujang honey sauce. Consume greedily and immediately.

Middle Eastern Spiced Salmon with Nutty Rice

Light Suppers

Diversity points: 8 / Fibre: 13g

4 salmon fillets

2 tsp sumac

1 tsp chilli flakes

1 tsp dried oregano

2 tbsp extra-virgin olive oil

Salt, to taste

FOR THE RICE

2 x 250g (9oz) pouches of pre-cooked grains or basmati and wild rice

150g (5oz/1 cup) pistachios (or cashews), roughly chopped

100g (3½oz)/⅔ cup toasted almonds, roughly chopped

150g (5oz/1 cup) dried apricots, roughly chopped

FOR THE SALAD

400g (14oz) cherry tomatoes, halved

200g (7oz) pomegranate seeds from a pack

2 tbsp extra-virgin olive oil

2 tsp pomegranate molasses (or balsamic vinegar)

+ Bonus Diversity Points

This dish would be lovely with a few balls of labneh from a jar, or even a large dollop of live Greek yoghurt. If you have fresh herbs to hand, add a handful to the rice along with a squeeze of lemon juice.

Those of you who have followed my cookery journey will know that this recipe is really very 'me'. It is a complete meal; from the deeply spiced, omega-rich crispy salmon to the nutty, buttery rice and zingy salad that pops with flavour and freshness. The recipe is infinitely adaptable so please do adjust to what you have available at home.

1. Once again to save time I use an air fryer, but you can just as easily fry the salmon in a non-stick frying pan drizzled with a little olive oil for 6-8 minutes. Put the salmon fillets skin side down into the air fryer and then sprinkle over the sumac, chilli flakes, oregano, and salt to taste. Drizzle over the olive oil and roast for 8–10 minutes at 200°C (400°F).

2. While the salmon is cooking, prepare your rice and salad. Follow the instructions on the packet to heat the rice in the microwave; once it has cooked through, toss into a bowl and add the chopped pistachios, almonds and apricots and season with a pinch of salt.

3. Put the cherry tomatoes into a bowl with the pomegranate seeds and dress with the olive oil and pomegranate molasses. Season with salt to taste.

4. Serve the salmon with the nutty rice and pomegranate and tomato salad alongside.

Time Saving Hack
When selecting salmon fillets, try and choose ones that are a little flatter and wider; this will save you a couple of minutes of cooking time.

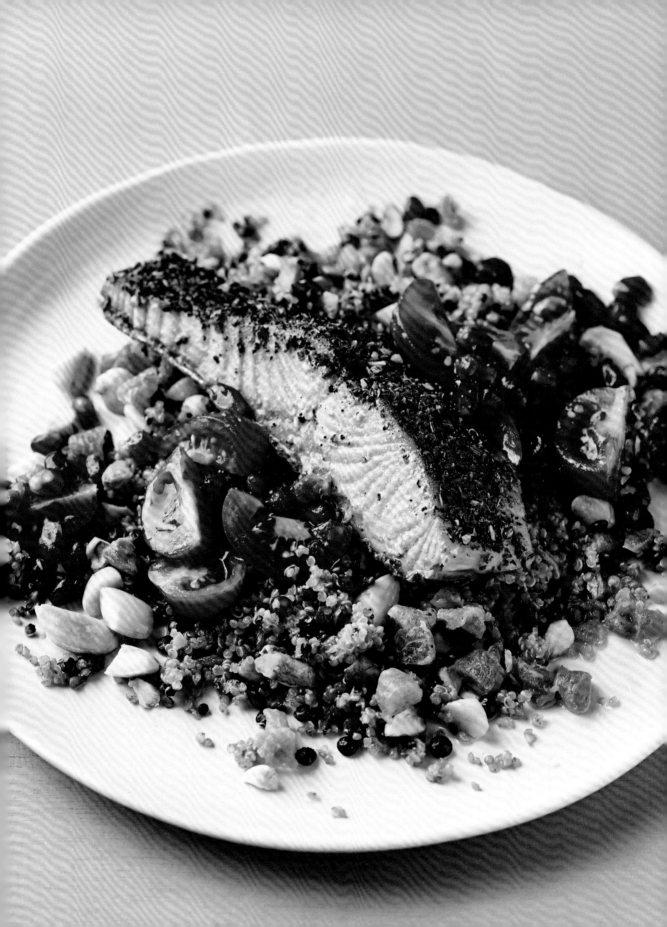

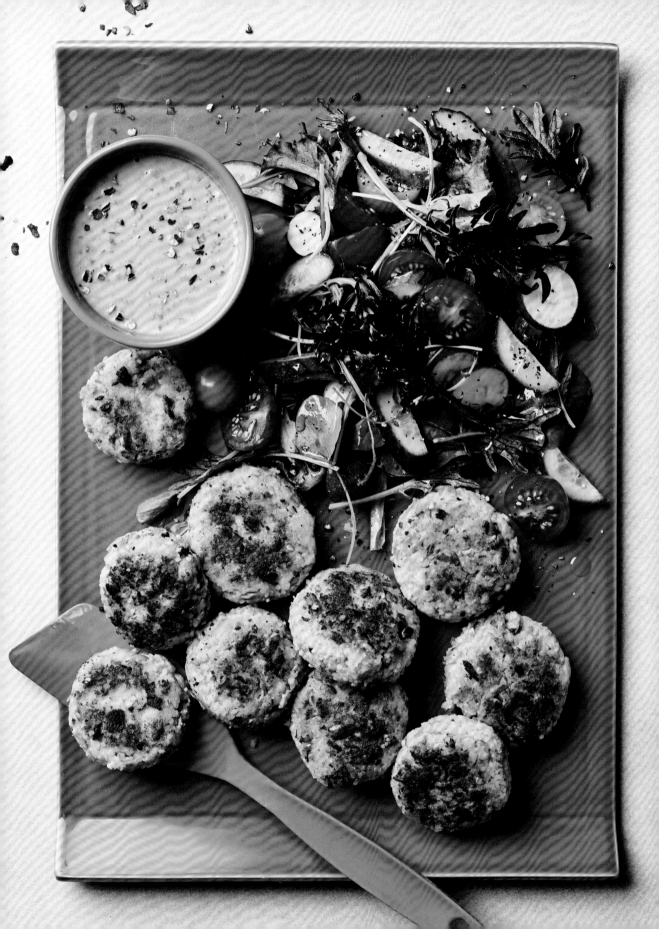

Tuna, Quinoa + Ginger Fishcakes with Peanut Sauce

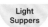

Light
Suppers

Diversity points: 6 / Fibre: 5.6g

400g (14oz) root veg mash (shop-bought, or home-made with potatoes, swedes, turnips)

2 x 145g (4½oz) tins tuna in spring water, drained

2 tsp ginger paste

1 tsp red chilli flakes

1 tsp lemongrass paste

250g (9oz) pouch of pre-cooked quinoa

1 tbsp vegetable oil

FOR THE SAUCE

2 tbsp heaped crunchy peanut better

2 tbsp soy sauce

2 tsp ginger paste

1 tbsp fish sauce

2 tsp honey

+ Bonus Diversity Points

Serve the fishcakes alongside some frozen broccoli and peas which have been cooked in the microwave.

Time Saving Hack

Root vegetable mash is available in most supermarkets. Its fibre content is higher than plain potato mash and it is a saviour, given how long root vegetables normally take to peel, cook and mash from scratch.

I love a fishcake but so many of the shop-bought varieties can be completely lacking in nutritional content. This one is enriched with root vegetable mash, lots of spices and quinoa. You can add even more vegetables to the fishcakes, for example chopped up cooked broccoli or cauliflower. I have even used these fishcakes inside burger buns, where they make a very worthy burger filling alongside a hot chilli sauce and lots of salad.

1. Tip the root vegetable mash into a large bowl and add the tuna, making sure that you've drained away all the liquid from the tin. Add the ginger, red chilli flakes, lemongrass paste and quinoa to the mixture and stir to combine. Portion the mixture out to make eight equal-sized fishcakes. The mixture should be fairly firm.

2. Place a non-stick frying pan over a medium heat and drizzle in the vegetable oil. When the oil is hot but not yet smoking, add the fishcakes to the pan – you'll likely need to cook these in two batches. Cook for about 2 minutes on each side; make sure you turn them with a fish slice and handle them gently so that they don't break. The idea is to create a nice golden crust.

3. While the fishcakes are cooking, combine all the ingredients for the sauce in a bowl along with a few tablespoons of kettle-hot water. Mix well to create a dipping sauce.

4. Serve the fishcakes alongside the dipping sauce and a salad of cherry tomatoes, cucumber, salad leaves and radish.

Braised Harissa Beans, Fennel + Orange Salad

Diversity points: 8 / Fibre: 23g

2 tbsp extra-virgin olive oil

1 tsp garlic paste

1 tsp mixed dried herbs

2 tbsp harissa paste

1 tsp nigella seeds

½ tsp fennel seeds

400g (14oz) tomato passata

1 x 400g (14oz) tin chickpeas

1 x 400g (14oz) tin butter beans

1 x 400g (14oz) tin black-eyed peas

Salt, to taste

FOR THE SALAD

2 fennel bulbs, thinly sliced

2 large oranges

2 tbsp extra-virgin olive oil

1 heaped tsp sumac

+ Bonus Diversity Points

Add finely diced onions, peppers, carrots and celery to the beans for extra plant diversity. Serve with any grains of your choice.

Time Saving Hack

Using passata is a fantastic way of saving time, just make sure you choose a variety with no added ingredients.

This recipe freezes really well so it's a great one to batch-cook and double up the quantities. Whenever I have defrosted beans from the freezer for dinner, I serve them alongside a fresh, citrussy salad, like the one I've given you here, to bring light and life to the dish. You can also serve with any grains of your choice or fibre-dense wholegrain bread.

1. Place a wide, flat casserole dish over a medium heat and drizzle in the olive oil. When the oil is hot but not quite smoking, add the garlic paste, dried herbs, harissa paste, nigella seeds and fennel seeds. Stir well until the spices are sizzling and start to release their aromas. At this point add the passata. Bring the mixture to the boil and allow it to reduce down for a couple of minutes until the rawness is cooked out of the passata.

2. Drain the chickpeas, butter beans and black-eyed peas in a colander and rinse through with some water. Transfer the beans to the casserole dish along with two-thirds of a tin of kettle-hot water. Let the mixture simmer, uncovered, for 10–12 minutes, stirring occasionally to ensure the beans don't catch. You want the beans to break down a little. Season with salt to taste.

3. While the beans are cooking, prepare the salad. Use a mandolin or sharp knife to cut the fennel into very thin slices or rounds. Peel the oranges, removing as much white pith as possible, then slice them horizontally into 1cm (½in) slices. Dress the fennel and orange with the extra-virgin olive oil and a touch of sumac for tartness and a tiny pinch of salt.

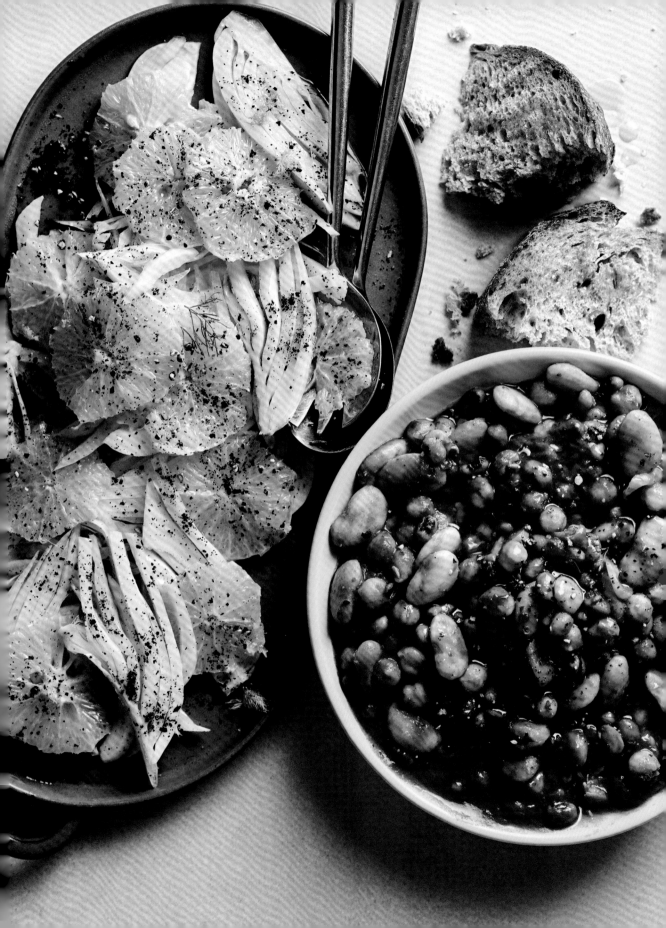

Masala Cod with Spiced Grains + Turmeric Yoghurt

Comforting Dinners

Diversity points: 6 / Fibre: 4.7g

2 tbsp vegetable oil

4 x 200g (7oz) skinless cod fillets

2 tsp red chilli powder

2 tsp ground cumin

1 tsp ground turmeric

Salt, to taste

FOR THE GRAINS

2 x 250g (9oz) pouches of pre-cooked mixed grains

4 tbsp light olive oil

2 tsp garlic paste

1 tsp cumin seeds

1 tsp mustard seeds

FOR THE SALAD

2 tomatoes, roughly chopped

1 red onion, roughly chopped

½ cucumber, roughly chopped

Juice of 1 lemon

1 tsp red chilli powder

Salt, to taste

FOR THE YOGHURT

250g (9oz) full-fat live Greek yoghurt

1 tsp ground turmeric

½ tsp black pepper

+ Bonus Diversity Points

By selecting a pouch of mixed grains you're ensuring that you optimise diversity. You can even add chickpeas or cooked lentils to the grains if you wish.

This is probably one of my signature dishes. Despite there being a couple of elements to pull together, it really is a very simple and time-efficient recipe. If you're not a fan of cod, then this recipe works well with a large chunk of paneer or thinly sliced chicken breast.

1. Place a non-stick frying pan over a medium heat and add the vegetable oil. Pat the cod dry with kitchen paper and dust evenly with the chilli powder, cumin and turmeric and season generously with salt. Use your fingers to rub the spices into the cod. Add the fish to the hot pan and fry for 2–3 minutes on each side until a deep golden crust forms on the surface and the flesh has just cooked through.

2. Heat the grains in the microwave following the packet instructions. While the grains are in the microwave, heat the olive oil in a saucepan and add the garlic, cumin and mustard seeds. As soon as they start to splutter, add the cooked grains from the pouch and stir well to combine. Remove from the heat.

3. For the salad and yoghurt simply combine the tomato, onion and cucumber in a bowl, squeeze over the lemon juice and season with salt and a touch of red chili powder. Combine the yoghurt, turmeric, black pepper and a touch of salt in another bowl, stirring well.

4. Spoon the grains on to four plates, top with the perfectly cooked cod and serve with the salad and yoghurt alongside.

 Time Saving Hack
Make sure your cod is no more than 3cm (1¼in thick to keep the cooking time down.

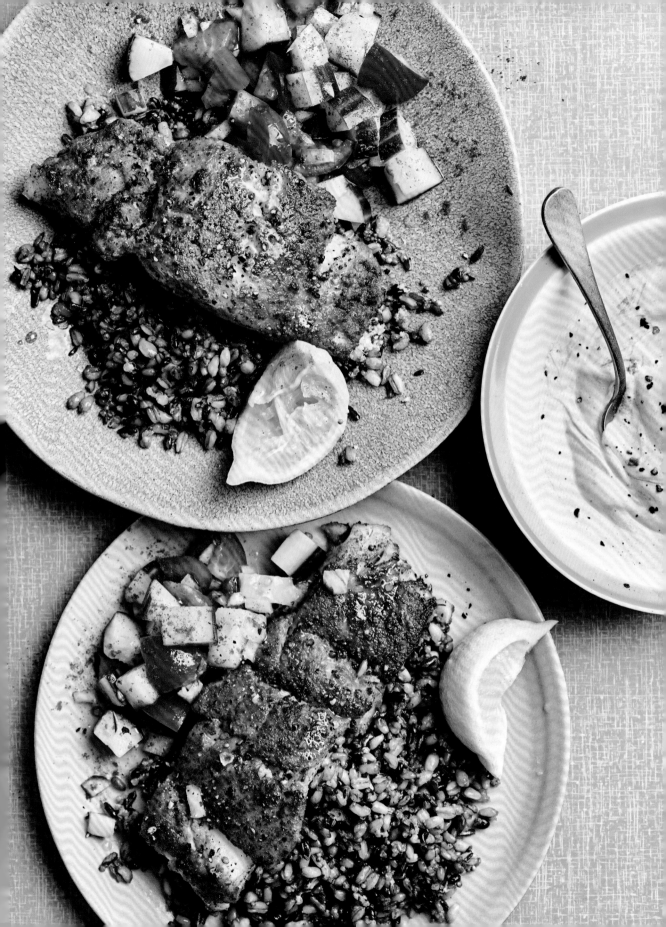

Chipotle Black Bean Soup with All The Toppings

Comforting Dinners

Diversity points: 6 / Fibre: 20g

2 tbsp extra-virgin olive oil

1 heaped tsp garlic paste

2 tbsp tomato purée

1 heaped tsp hot paprika

2 tsp chipotle paste

3 x 400g (14oz) tins black beans, drained

750ml (1¼ pints/3 cups) kettle-hot water or hot vegetable stock

Salt, to taste

FOR THE TOPPINGS

2 tomatoes, diced

½ red onion, diced

Juice of 1 lime

1 large or 2 small avocados,

4 tbsp full-fat live Greek yoghurt

2 red or green chillies, thinly sliced

125g (4oz) feta cheese, crumbled

75g (2¾oz) maize or blue corn tortilla chips

+ Bonus Diversity Points

If you have time, finely dice carrots, celery and peppers and sweat them down at the start of the recipe before adding the spices.

Time Saving Hack
I would highly recommend you invest in a stick blender; they are cheap and you don't need a high-quality one. It saves having to transfer the hot beans to a blender and from the blender back into the saucepan.

This soup has so many accompaniments that it hardly feels like a soup anymore. I love bringing the extra toppings to the table where everybody can load on their favourites; chipotle paste and extra paprika give the soup real oomph. If you have any home-made stock or bone broth, then use this instead of water for added to depth of flavour.

1. Start by putting a kettle full of water on to boil. Add the extra-virgin olive oil and garlic to a saucepan and place over a medium heat. When the garlic starts to sizzle, add the tomato purée and cook out the rawness for a minute. Then add the paprika, chipotle paste and the drained black beans. Stir well to combine everything, then pour in the water or stock.

2. Let the mixture simmer for a couple of minutes, then use a stick blender to blitz into a soup. I like a slightly chunky consistency, but you can go for a smooth soup if you prefer. Adjust the consistency of the soup with more liquid, depending on how you like it.

3. While the soup is simmering, prepare all your toppings. Combine the diced tomato and red onion in a bowl and squeeze over half the lime juice. Remove the stone from the avocado and cut the flesh into slices, then squeeze over the other lime half to stop the avocado browning.

4. Ladle the soup into bowls and top with Greek yoghurt, then let everyone add their own toppings: diced tomato and onion, avocado slices, sliced chillies, crumbled feta and crushed tortilla chips for added crunch.

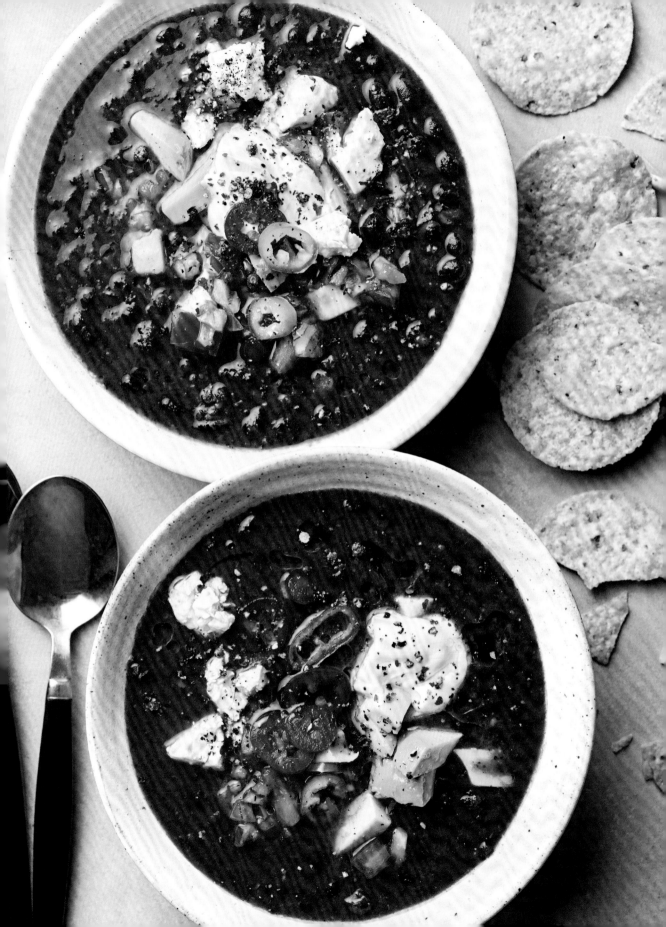

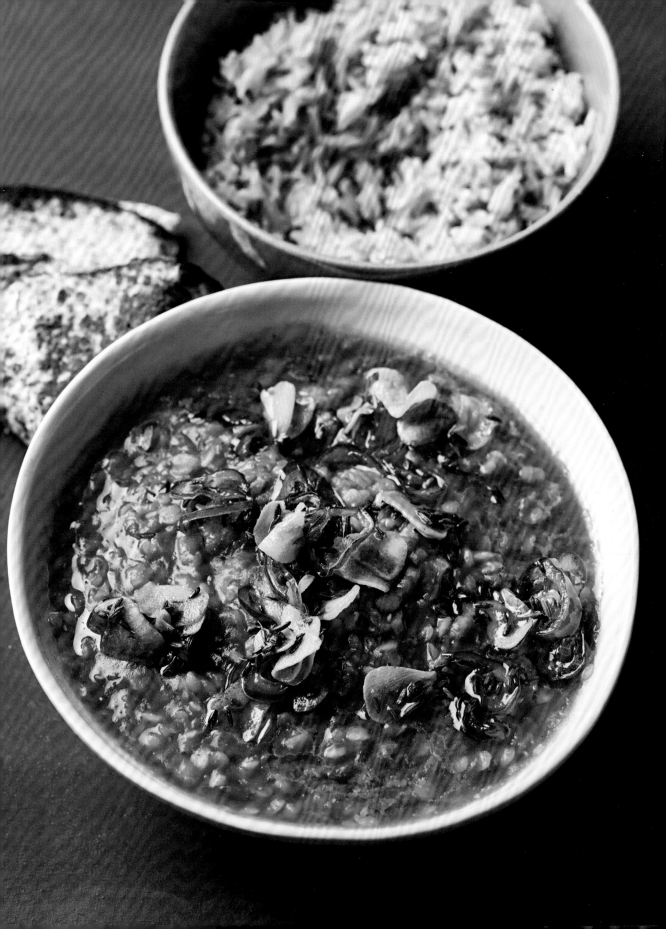

Microwave Lentils with Chilli Cumin Oil

Comforting Dinners

Diversity points: 4 / Fibre: 9.9g

125g (4oz) red lentils
½ x 400g (14oz) tin chopped tomatoes
½ tsp ground turmeric
1 tsp red chilli powder
550ml (18fl oz/2 cups) kettle-hot water
2 tbsp olive oil or ghee
2 garlic cloves, thinly sliced
1 green chilli, thinly sliced
1 tsp cumin seeds
Salt, to taste
Wholewheat chapattis or rice, to serve

+ Bonus Diversity Points

Add a tin of chickpeas or other pulse of your choice to the red lentils. You can also wilt some fresh spinach leaves into the daal when it comes out piping hot from the microwave. Add lots of herbs like dill and coriander and serve with a side salad.

It's no exaggeration when I say that my life changed the day I discovered that I could make daal from scratch in 12 minutes in a microwave. It gives me great pleasure to impart this wisdom on to you. If you are able to soak the lentils beforehand this will improve the texture of the daal even more, but it certainly isn't a prerequisite.

1. Pour the red lentils and chopped tomatoes into a large microwave-safe bowl which has a tight-fitting lid. Add the turmeric and chilli powder followed by the hot water. Stir well to combine, then cover the bowl with the lid and microwave for 12-15 minutes. If your microwave-safe bowl doesn't have a lid, you can also wrap tightly with clingfilm.

2. While the daal is in the microwave, heat the olive oil or ghee in a small saucepan. Add the garlic, green chilli and cumin seeds and cook gently until the garlic turns golden.

3. Remove the daal from the microwave and very carefully take off the lid (a lot of steam will release rapidly and it can burn). Take a fork and use it to mix the daal really well, then season with salt to taste.

4. Pour the hot, spiced garlicky oil over the daal and serve immediately with warmed chapattis or rice.

Time Saving Hack
Note that it takes approximately 30 minutes to cook red lentils on the stove and you will need to stir fairly frequently. This microwave daal technique cuts cooking time by more than half.

Tandoori Chickpeas + Gingery Sweet Potatoes with Mango Chutney Raita

Comforting Dinners

Diversity points: 5 / Fibre: 22g

1 tbsp olive oil	
1 tsp garlic paste	
2 generous tbsp tandoori marinade paste	
2 x 400g (14oz) tins chickpeas, drained and rinsed	
Thumb-sized piece of ginger, peeled and julienned	
1 red or green chilli, thinly sliced	
½ red onion, thinly sliced	
4 large, pre-roasted sweet potatoes	
4 tbsp full-fat live Greek yoghurt	
2 tbsp mango chutney	
Salt, to taste	

+ Bonus Diversity Points
Serve with a side salad, or you can top with extra nuts and seeds e.g. toasted peanuts and pumpkin seeds to add texture.

Time Saving Hack
Try and select a tandoori marinade paste that doesn't have added food colouring, emulsifiers, preservatives etc. Tandoori paste isn't mandatory – you can also use a good curry powder or jalfrezi/ korma paste.

A recipe that'll make you go 'phwoar'. The real time-saving hack here is to have the sweet potatoes pre-roasted and ready in the fridge, so that all you have to do is heat them up in the microwave and load them with the tandoori chickpea filling.

1. Put a kettle full of water on to boil.

2. Heat the olive oil in a saucepan over a medium heat and add the garlic paste. When the garlic starts to sizzle add the tandoori marinade paste and stir well to cook out the rawness. Add the chickpeas to the pan and stir well to combine, using the back of the spoon to break down some of the chickpeas. Add about 150ml (5fl oz/⅔ cup) of kettle-hot water to the chickpea mixture and simmer for a couple of minutes until they are jammy and thick. Season with salt to taste.

3. While the chickpeas are simmering away prepare the ginger, chilli and red onion.

4. Microwave the sweet potatoes for about 2 minutes so they're piping hot, then slice them in half and load them with the chickpeas. Top with yoghurt and mango chutney followed by the sliced ginger, chilli and onion.

+ Note
If you have time, you can pan fry the ginger in a tablespoon of vegetable oil until it is slightly golden and crisp. This makes the ginger even tastier.

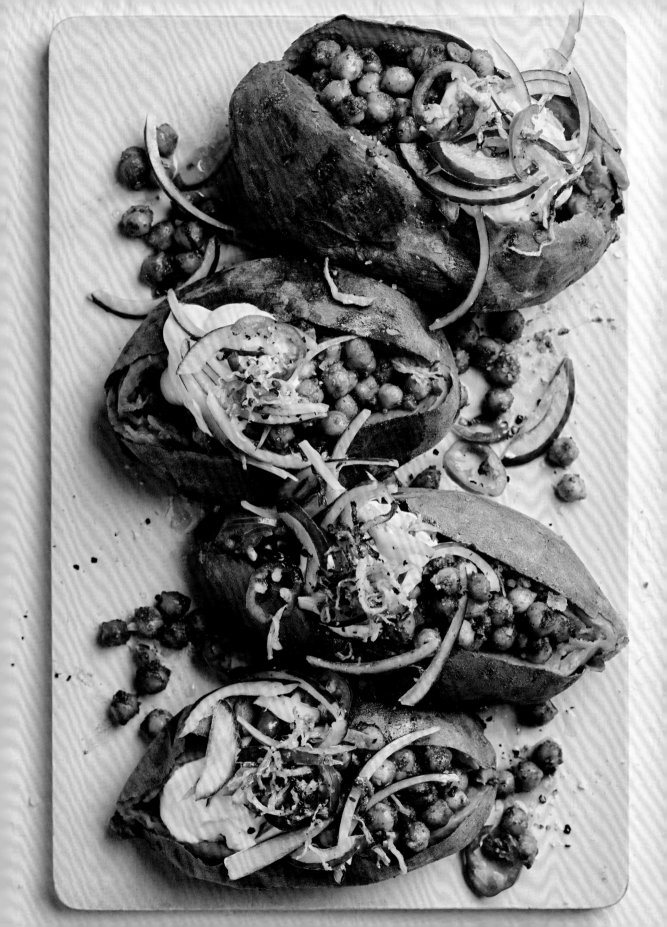

Creamy Leeks + Cannellini Beans with Za'atar

Comforting Dinners

Diversity points: 5 / Fibre: 15g (including pitta)

2 tbsp extra-virgin olive oil, plus extra for drizzling

300g (10oz) leeks, finely chopped

1 tsp garlic paste

Few sprigs of thyme, leaves picked

2 x 400g (14oz) tins cannellini beans, drained

50g (2oz/½ cup) jumbo oats

600ml (20fl oz/2½ cups) boiling hot water or stock

4 tbsp full-fat live yoghurt

4 tsp za'atar

Handful of roughly chopped parsley

Grated Parmesan cheese (*optional*)

Salt and pepper, to taste

Toasted pitta or seedy crackers, to serve

+ Bonus Diversity Points

You can add any leftover grains to the stew. If you want to go a little bit greener why not wilt through some spinach, kale and/or spring greens?

Time Saving Hack

I often buy my vegetables from the sales section in the supermarket where vegetables near their sell-by date are to be found. Pre-chopped leeks packaged in small plastic bags feature regularly here. You may need to cook them that evening, but I often use them to make this dish as leftovers can be frozen for another day.

Velvety, brothy stews made with softened leeks and tender cannellini beans have been popping up on various food blogs and social media platforms and, in my opinion, the hype is well deserved. Not only does this recipe take minutes to come together, it gives the illusion that the beans have been bubbling away for hours on the stove. My version has the addition of oats, which are a fantastic source of soluble fibre and also thicken the dish beautifully.

1. Put a kettle full of water on to boil. Heat the olive oil in a saucepan over a medium heat and add the leeks. Allow them to soften for 2–3 minutes, then add the garlic paste and thyme followed by the cannellini beans and oats. I tend to drain the excess water from the tinned beans but not rinse them as the residual aquafaba helps thicken the final dish.

2. Add the kettle-hot water (or stock if you have it) to the beans and season liberally with salt and pepper. Allow the mixture to boil vigorously and thicken for 5 minutes, stirring regularly.

3. Ladle the beans into bowls and top with a dollop of live yoghurt, a healthy drizzle of olive oil and a good sprinkling of za'atar and some chopped parsley. Sometimes, when I don't have yoghurt, I finish the dish with a flourish of Parmesan for extra umami goodness. I prefer this dish on its own without any sides, but you can try it with toasted pitta bread or seedy crackers if you wish.

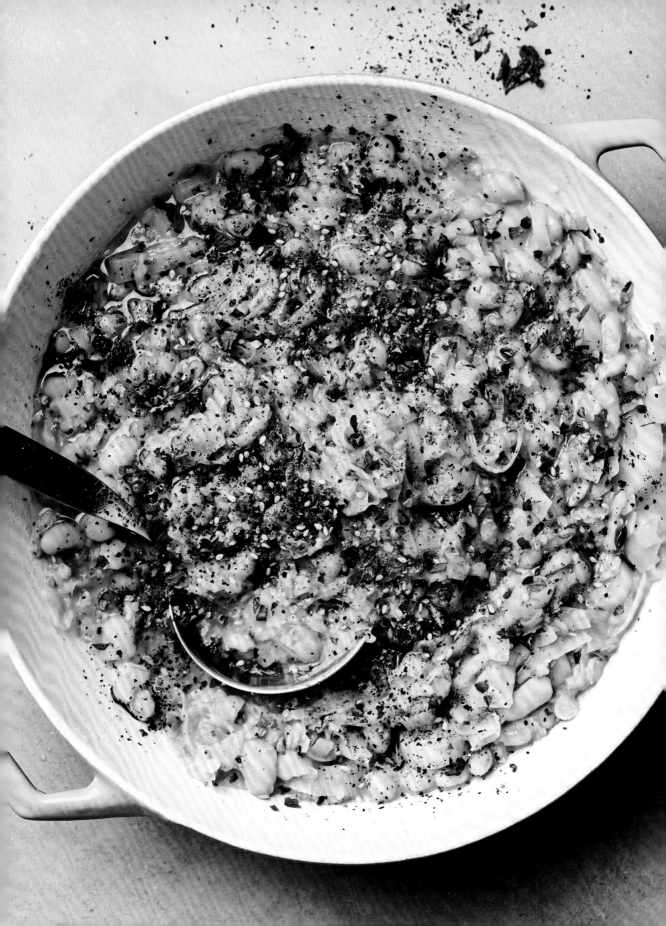

Sour Red Pepper + Peanut Curry

Comforting
Dinners

Diversity points: 7 / Fibre: 10g

3 tbsp vegetable oil
1 heaped tsp ginger paste
½ tsp fennel seeds
1 tsp cumin seeds
½ tsp caraway seeds
½–1 tsp red chilli powder
2 red peppers, deseeded and thickly sliced
1 green pepper, deseeded and thickly sliced
1 yellow pepper, deseeded and thickly sliced
3 heaped tbsp tamarind chutney
100g (3½oz/⅔ cup) toasted peanuts
Salt, to taste
Toasted flatbreads e.g. pitta or naan bread, to serve

+ Bonus Diversity Points

Add tomatoes and onions to the peppers if you wish.

A flavoursome dry curry which can be enjoyed with flatbreads. To save time I use shop-bought tamarind chutney but you can soak your own tamarind pulp in water and use this with some maple syrup instead. If you're looking to up your protein consumption you may wish to add some lightly fried chunks of paneer cheese. The spices I have used are an aromatic mixture, but feel free to add your favourites.

1. Place a wide, non-stick frying pan over a medium-high heat. Add the vegetable oil to the pan followed by the ginger paste, fennel, cumin and caraway seeds and red chilli powder and fry, stirring.

2. When the spices have released their aromas, add the peppers and stir-fry for 2–3 minutes before adding the tamarind chutney and half a mugful of kettle-hot water. Season with salt to taste. Allow the sauce to reduce down for a few minutes before topping with the toasted peanuts.

3. Serve with toasted flatbreads.

Time Saving Hack
Rather than slicing the peppers in half and then removing the seeds, place the pepper on your chopping board and use your thumb to press down on the stalk. This will detach the seeds in one go and save you time.

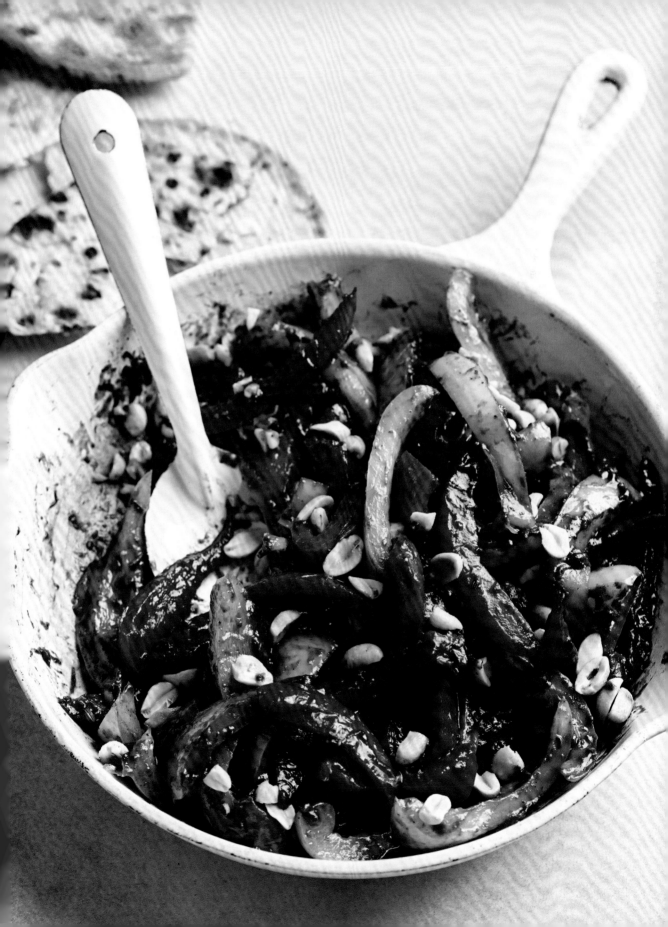

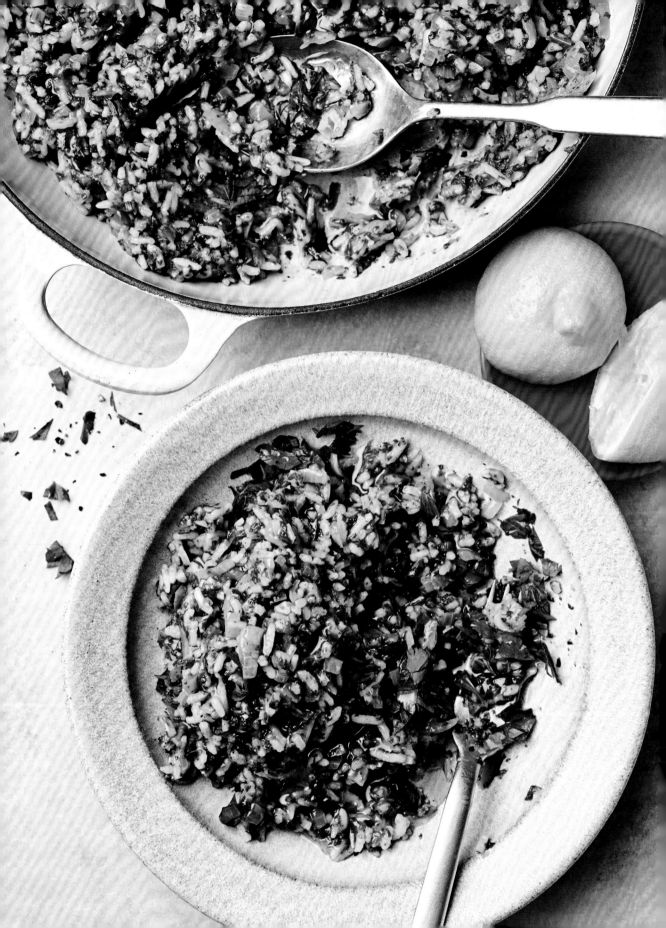

Greek-Inspired Lemony Spinach + Rice

Comforting
Dinners

Diversity points: 5 / Fibre: 3.5g

4 tbsp extra-virgin olive oil

6 garlic cloves

400g (14oz) frozen chopped onion

2 tsp dried oregano

2 tsp chilli flakes

600g (1lb 5oz) frozen chopped spinach

2 x 250g (9oz) pouches of pre-cooked short-grain rice

450ml (16fl oz/1¾ cups) hot stock or kettle-hot water

Juice of 1–2 lemons

Handful of parsley leaves, roughly torn

+ Bonus Diversity Points
Sauté the onions with leeks and add a few large handfuls of finely chopped dill.

One pan, a bit of spinach, rice and lemon. That's virtually all you need in this recipe. I find myself craving this dish often as it is so simple but exceptionally moreish. The addition of lemon juice to spinach actually enhances the absorption of iron in the gut, so it's a win-win all round.

1. Put a kettle of water on to boil. Place a casserole dish over a medium heat and drizzle in the olive oil; when the olive oil is hot but not yet smoking, add the garlic and sauté until it starts to turn golden. Add the chopped onion, oregano and chilli flakes and stir well. Sauté for a further 2–3 minutes to allow the excess moisture from the onions to evaporate and for them to soften slightly.

2. While the onions are cooking, defrost the spinach in a microwave for about 2½ minutes, then add to the softened onions and stir well. Crumble the rice from the pouches into the spinach and top with the hot stock or water. Stir well and allow the rice and spinach to simmer for 3–4 more minutes until most of the moisture has evaporated. Squeeze in the lemon juice before serving and scatter over the parsley.

 ### Time Saving Hack
To save you time, this recipe uses not one, not two, but three time-saving ingredients: frozen chopped spinach, frozen chopped onions and pre-cooked short-grain rice.

Harissa Apricot Chicken Kebabs

Comforting Dinners

Diversity points: 6 / Fibre: 9.4g

| |
400g (14oz) diced chicken thighs

2 spring onions, roughly chopped

2 heaped tbsp rose harissa paste

15g (1oz) parsley or coriander

6 dried apricots

Flatbreads, to serve (optional)

THE SALAD

¼ white cabbage (about 200g/7oz), finely shredded

5 dried apricots, roughly chopped

Handful of parsley leaves, finely chopped

1–2 tbsp apple cider vinegar

1 tbsp extra-virgin olive oil

1 x 400g (14oz) tin green lentils, drained and rinsed

Salt, to taste

FOR THE YOGHURT

250g (9oz) full-fat live Greek yoghurt

1 tbsp rose harissa paste

1 tbsp extra-virgin olive oil

+ Bonus Diversity Points
Serve this dish alongside a selection of lacto-fermented pickles in brine.

Time Saving Hack
Using a food processor cuts down on prep time and you won't get your hands dirty when making the mixture. Consider leaving it on the worktop so you are ready to get started in the evening.

I think it's near enough impossible for me to write a book without including a kebab recipe. The intense piquant tone of harissa matches the tannin sweetness of apricots, a marriage made in heaven. For the accompanying salad, cabbage is a more nutritious alternative to lettuce, given it is a prebiotic brassica.

1. Put the chicken, spring onions, harissa, parsley or coriander and dried apricots into a food processor and blitz to form a consistency similar to sausage meat.

2. Place a non-stick frying pan over a medium heat. Divide the kebab mixture into six portions. Spoon each portion into the frying pan, flattening it with a back of a spoon to make roughly circular or oval kebabs which are no more than 1cm (½in) thick and 10cm (4in) wide. Fry the kebabs for about 2–3 minutes on each side.

3. While the kebabs are frying, prepare all your salad ingredients. Mix the cabbage, apricots and parsley in a bowl with the vinegar and extra-virgin olive oil to make a quick salad. Season to taste with salt. Transfer the lentils to a microwave-safe bowl and microwave for 2 minutes before spreading them out over a platter. Toss the cabbage salad over these warm lentils.

4. Put the Greek yoghurt into a bowl and marble in the harissa paste and extra-virgin olive oil through it.

5. Serve the kebabs with the lentil, cabbage and apricot salad and the marbled harissa yoghurt alongside.

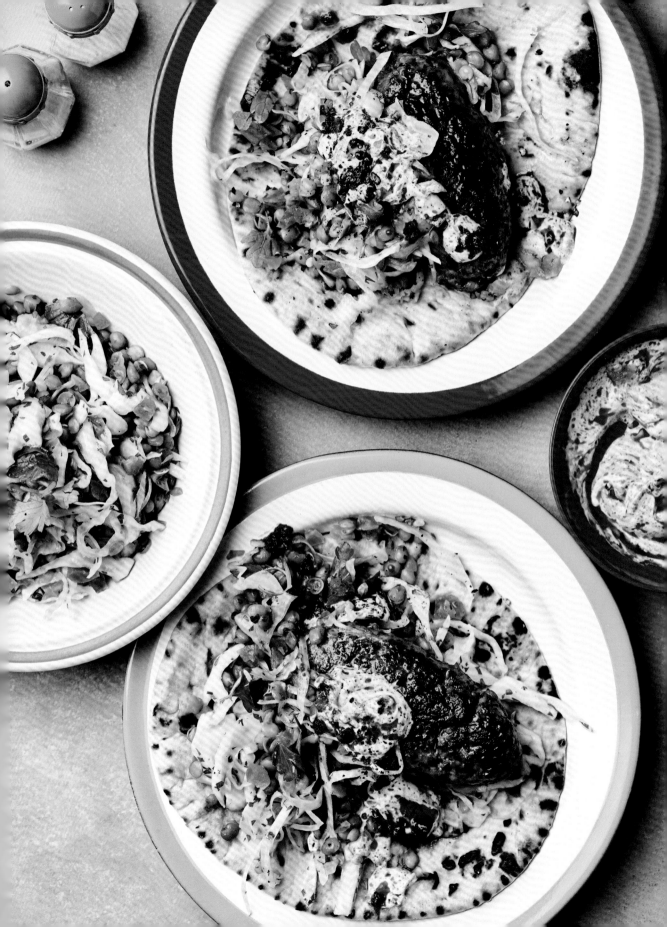

Emerald Pasta

Comforting
Dinners

Diversity points: 5 / Fibre: 7.9g

| 250g (9oz) ditalini or macaroni pasta |
| 150g (5oz) cavolo nero |
| 30g (1oz) dill |
| 30g (1oz) coriander |
| 1 x 400g (14oz) tin chickpeas |
| 2 small or 1 large garlic clove |
| Juice of ½ lemon |
| Generous drizzle extra-virgin olive oil |
| 2 tbsp grated Parmesan cheese (optional) |
| Salt and pepper, to taste |

+ Bonus Diversity Points
You can use tinned black-eyed peas, white beans and green lentils instead of chickpeas or add extra frozen peas if you wish.

Cavolo nero, with its slightly bitter undertones, is paired with creamy chickpeas to make a vivid emerald pasta sauce. This is one of those recipes that you will find yourself turning to time and time again. It is both deeply comforting and virtuous in equal measure. Feel free to switch the cavolo nero for spring greens, kale, spinach or rocket leaves.

1. Put a kettle full of hot water on to boil, then pour the boiling water into a saucepan and add the pasta and a generous amount of salt. Cook over a medium heat according to the packet instructions.

2. While the pasta is cooking, strip the cavolo nero leaves off the stalks and place them in a microwave-safe bowl. Splash with a little water, cover the bowl and microwave on high heat for about 3 minutes. Transfer the cavolo nero to a blender along with the dill, coriander, half of the chickpeas, about half of the aquafaba from the tin and the garlic. Season with salt and pepper and blitz to a smooth purée.

3. Drain the pasta, reserving a little of the pasta water. Return the pasta to the pan and add the green sauce from the blender, along with the remaining chickpeas and the lemon juice. Return to a medium heat, add a splash of the reserved pasta water and simmer for a minute or two. Taste and adjust the seasonings if you wish, then drizzle with extra-virgin olive oil. I also like to serve with a little grated Parmesan over the top.

Time Saving Hack
Use a shape of pasta that has a short cooking time, like macaroni, orzo or ditalini.

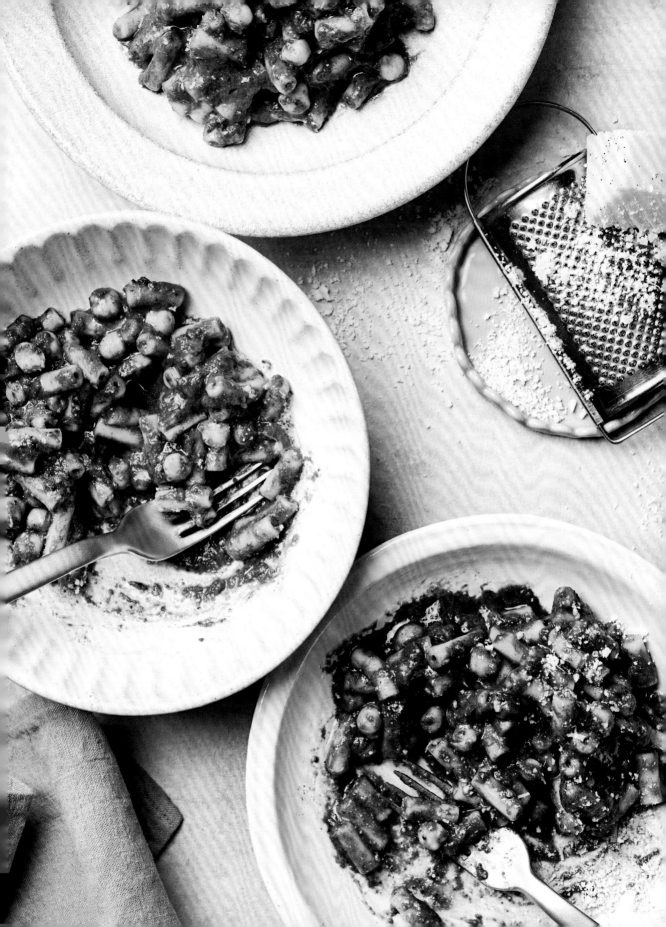

Moroccan-Inspired Lamb with Carrot + Date Couscous

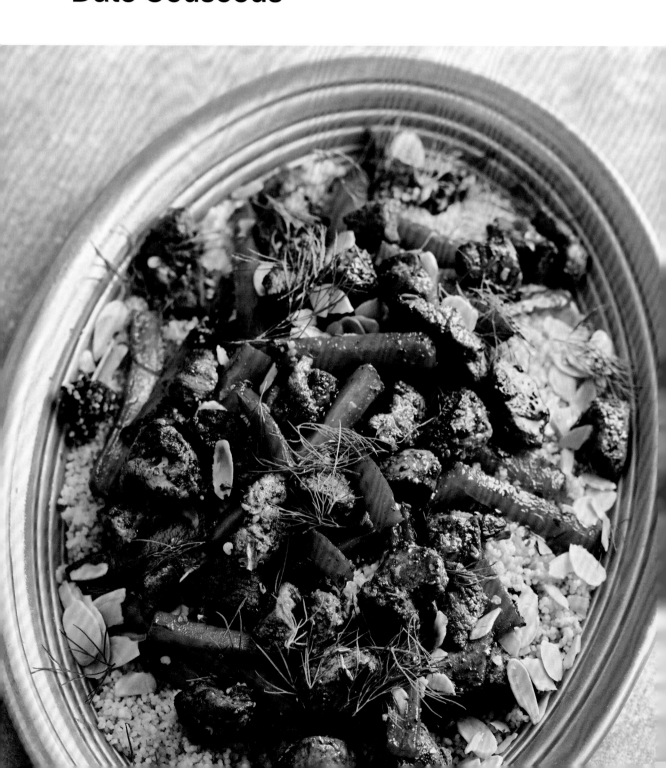

Diversity points: 6 / Fibre: 10g

200g (7oz/1 cup) couscous

Juice of 1 lemon

300g (10oz) pre-cut carrot batons

1 tbsp extra-virgin olive oil

1 tsp honey

½–1 tsp chilli flakes

4 dates, stoned

300g (10oz) boneless lamb, cut into 1cm (½in) cubes

2 tsp ras el hanout

2 tsp garlic paste

1 tbsp vegetable oil

Salt, to taste

OPTIONAL TOPPINGS

Toasted almonds

Chopped dill

Crumbled feta

+ Bonus Diversity Points

Add chickpeas or other lentils/beans of your choice to the couscous.

Time Saving Hack

Make sure you select an instant couscous which has a very short cooking time. Using a spice blend like ras el hanout is preferable to spending ages adding multiple different spices from your cupboard. I use ready prepared carrot batons in this recipe, but you can simply peel and slice the carrots into chunky rounds if you prefer.

A perfumed, exotic dish: close your eyes and you will be transported deep into the depths of a Moroccan souk. Ras el hanout is a popular Moroccan spice blend that is a staple in my store cupboard. It reminds me of a mellow garam masala and gives this dish slow-cooked tagine vibes, when in reality it has come together in minutes.

1. Bring a kettle of water to the boil. Put the couscous into a bowl and top with the boiling water so it rises about 1cm (½in) above the surface of the couscous. Squeeze in the lemon juice and add a pinch of salt, then cover with a tight-fitting lid and allow to sit for 10 minutes.

2. Meanwhile, put the carrots into a saucepan with 3 tablespoons of water and place over a medium-high heat to steam for a couple of minutes until most of the water has evaporated. Add the olive oil, honey and chilli flakes and cook for 2–3 minutes more, stirring well to coat the carrots and caramelise them slightly. Remove from the heat and allow to cool. Chop or tear the dates into the carrot mixture.

3. Put the lamb, ras el hanout and garlic into a bowl and stir to combine. Heat the vegetable oil in a large non-stick frying pan over a high heat; when the oil is almost smoking, add the lamb and brown on all sides. You are looking to achieve a golden crust on all sides of the lamb, so a high heat is essential. If the temperature isn't high enough the meat will stew instead of caramelise. It will take just 2–3 last minutes for the lamb to cook through; cooking for much longer will result in tough meat.

4. Uncover the couscous, fluff up the grains with a fork and transfer to a large platter. Top the couscous with the carrot and date mixture followed by the lamb. Add any of the optional toppings that you have in your store cupboard or fridge and serve immediately.

Marry-Me Red Pasta

Comforting Dinners

Diversity points: 5 / Fibre: 9.2g

250g (9oz) spaghetti

175g (6oz) sun-dried tomatoes and 2 tbsp of their oil

300g (10oz) cherry tomatoes

75g (2¾oz) pitted black olives

175g (6oz) jarred peppers (ideally in light vinegar or brine)

1 tbsp pomegranate molasses

1 tsp red chilli flakes

2–3 garlic cloves (or 1 heaped tsp garlic paste)

1 tbsp extra-virgin olive oil, plus extra for drizzling

200g (7oz) raw, shelled, deveined prawns

2 tbsp grated Parmesan cheese (optional)

Salt, to taste

Rocket leaves dressed with lemon juice, to serve (optional)

+ Bonus Diversity Points
You can brown a chopped onion to form the base of the tomato sauce or add a handful of herbs such as dill and parsley to the final dish.

Time Saving Hack
The combination of sun-dried tomatoes, roasted peppers and pomegranate molasses gives a real intensity to the sauce, so you don't even realise that it is a 'no cook' recipe. Choose a spaghetti that has a short boil time. Slightly thinner strands of spaghetti can often cook in half the time.

This is a romantic recipe that is perfect for a date night at home. The red pasta sauce is 'no cook' – the blender does the work so you don't have to. My only absolute is that you use good-quality, sweet cherry tomatoes that don't taste watery or bland. Cherry tomatoes should be perfumed and a rich red colour; even better, on the vine.

1. Boil a kettle full of water, then pour the boiling water into a large saucepan and place over a high heat. Add the spaghetti and a generous amount of salt and cook until al dente, according to the instructions on the packet. Drain the pasta, reserving a little pasta water.

2. Add the sun-dried tomatoes and some of the sun-dried tomato oil to a blender with the cherry tomatoes, black olives, roasted red peppers, pomegranate molasses, chilli flakes and garlic and top up with two ladles full of the pasta water. Blitz to a smooth purée.

3. Add the extra-virgin olive oil to the same pan that the pasta was cooked in and warm through the prawns for just a minute – you don't want them to go chewy and tough. Pour the tomato sauce from the blender over the prawns and season with a little salt to taste. Stir well, then add the pasta and stir again until the sauce has coated the pasta. Transfer to bowls and drizzle over some extra olive oil and Parmesan cheese (if using). I like to serve alongside some rocket leaves dressed with lemon juice.

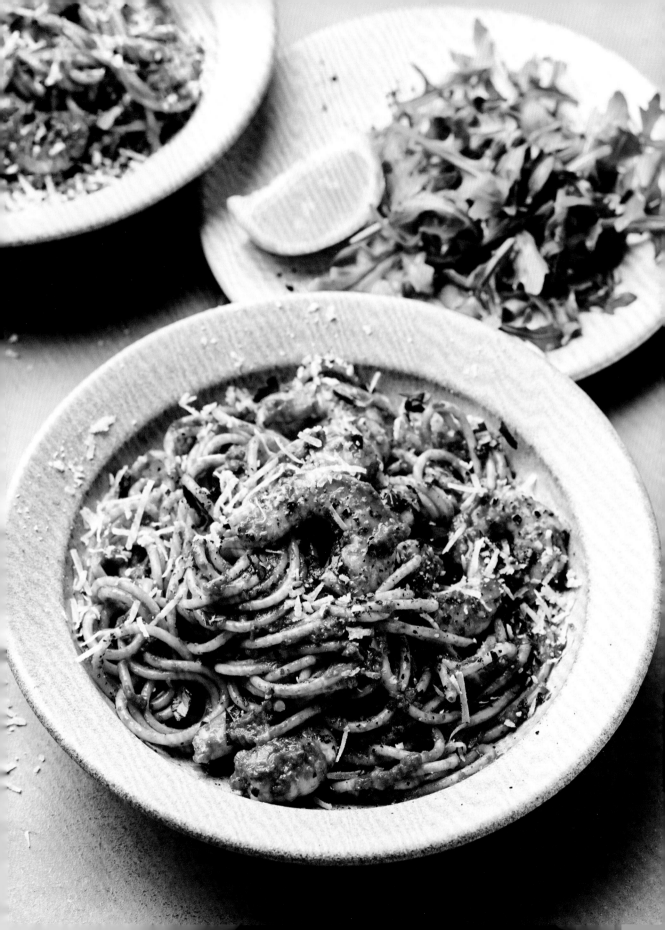

Cheesy One-Pot Orzo with Greens

Comforting
Dinners

Diversity points: 4 / Fibre: 8.7g

350g (12oz) orzo

1 litre (1¾ pints/4 cups) hot vegetable or chicken stock

2 tsp garlic paste

350g (12oz) broccoli (1 small or ½ large head of broccoli)

100g (3½oz) frozen garden peas

100g (3½oz) frozen shelled broad beans

250g (9oz) crème fraîche

150g (5½oz) mature Cheddar cheese, grated

4 tbsp Parmesan or vegetarian hard cheese

1 tsp cracked black pepper

Salt, to taste

+ Bonus Diversity Points

Add frozen spinach and finely chopped parsley if you wish. Sun-dried tomatoes can also add a burst of flavour. Serve alongside a salad of rocket leaves dressed with lemon juice and if you like a bit of crunch, some stale breadcrumbs fried in olive oil with lemon zest would make a superb topping.

A cheesy, unctuous pasta dish that brings much-needed comfort in times of need. Thankfully it all comes together in one pot, so there's very little in the way of washing up, plus it should be an instant hit with the children. It will taste better if you have any home-made stock to hand, if not, just use an organic stock cube of your choice dissolved in water.

1. Put the orzo into a large, shallow cast-iron pan, add the hot stock and garlic paste and place over a medium-high heat. Stir well and let the mixture bubble away for 4–5 minutes, stirring occasionally to make sure the orzo doesn't stick to the base of the pan.

2. Meanwhile, chop the broccoli into small florets. Add the broccoli to the orzo along with the garden peas and broad beans. It will take the vegetables a further 4–5 minutes to cook through. You will need to keep stirring the pot to prevent the orzo from sticking. You are aiming for a risotto like consistency.

3. Once the vegetables and orzo are cooked through, remove from the heat and add the crème fraîche, Cheddar and Parmesan and stir really well to combine everything. Finish with a really generous amount of black pepper and a touch of salt if you need it (stock and cheese can often be quite salty, so exercise caution). Serve immediately.

Time Saving Hack
I use orzo to save time as it cooks very quickly. You may wish to use macaroni instead.

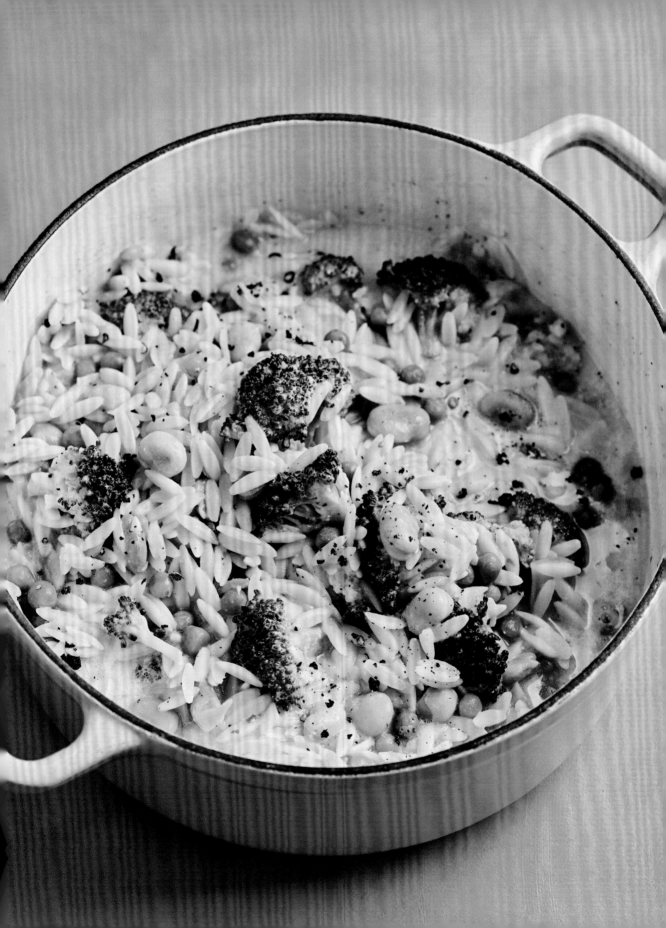

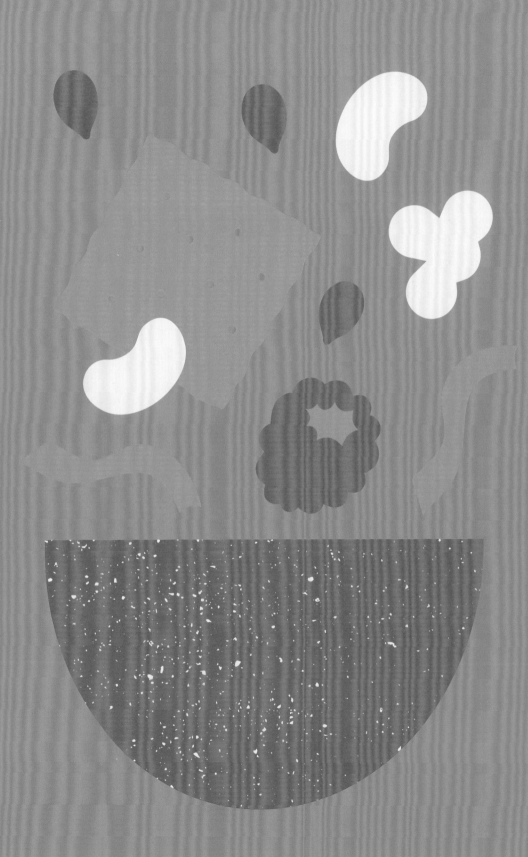

Snack Attack

chapter five

When was the last time you went a day without snacking? Last week? Last month? Last year? Never? For me, in a family of two busy doctors raising two energetic boys, sometimes it feels like snacks are the only things keeping us afloat, and I imagine many of you readers have experienced a similar dynamic.

Across the world, snacking habits have increased exponentially over the last few decades. Next time you are in the supermarket have a look at how much shelf space is dedicated to snacks in all their various forms, compared to the amount of space given to fresh fruit or vegetables, and you'll understand the scale of the pressure.

If I could give you one piece of advice it would be this: beware of the 'health halo'. Snacks that look healthy – and are often marketed as such – can be filled with all manner of hidden nasties; for example, low-fat fruit yoghurts loaded with sweeteners, additives and preservatives. Or some quinoa, chickpea and vegetable puffs that contain huge amounts of salt, fat and remain ultra-processed food items.

Although I personally prefer eating at prescribed mealtimes, I often find that my brain is trying its hardest to convince my body that it needs a boost of energy without which it would surely wither away into nothing. Because snacking can be closely linked to our underlying subconscious emotional state, any change in behaviour requires us to first understand that behaviour more fully. If you asked yourself, every time you reached into the snack cupboard, why your hand was in there, what would the answer be? If you're anything like me, the answer will be different each time you head for a snack. It might be boredom, anxiety,

loneliness, fatigue or a skipped meal, or maybe it's a mental crutch that your brain has become accustomed to before it can unwind and relax? I often observe patients 'stress snacking', where the snack item, usually sugary or carb-heavy items like biscuits, crisps and soft drinks, are used to distract or combat the negative effects of the stress they are experiencing.

Alongside the why of snacking is also the when? Do you snack at a set time every day, or is it more erratic and unpredictable? Are you trapped in a 'starve and stuff' cycle, where a skipped lunch is replaced by a mountain of snacks around 3pm? Do you find it difficult to pass a vending machine or a newsagent on your break without checking your pocket for change? Or do you snack after your evening meal in front of the TV? For me it's clear that only when we understand the why and when of snacking can we start to change the what.

So, how do we avoid these seemingly unavoidable snacking pitfalls? Perhaps keep a snack diary for a week or two and if possible, recognise, schedule and prepare in advance snacks for points of the day where you need an extra boost? Ten to fifteen minutes a week of bulk-preparation can help you to snack mindfully and healthily, safe in the knowledge that you know exactly what is going into your body. What's more, the recipes in this chapter are full of fibre, designed to keep you feeling full for longer, and not a single ingredient begins with the letter E followed by a number!

Transform your snacks from sugar, salt and guilt into goodness and intention. Happy snacking!

Tropical Trail Mix

Diversity points: 8 / Fibre: 4.7g

75g (2¾oz/¾ cup) freeze-dried banana chips

75g (2¾oz/½ cup) dried mango

75g (2¾oz/¾ cup) dried goji berries

100g (3½oz/1 cup) pecans

100g (3½oz/1 cup) hazelnuts

50g (2oz/⅔ cup) pumpkin seeds

25g (1oz/½ cup) dried coconut chips

100g (3½oz/⅔ cup) dried apricots (avoid ones that are very soft/moist)

+ Bonus Diversity Points

There are an endless number of dried fruits or nuts that you could add to this diversity mix. A general pointer would be to opt for varieties of dried fruit that don't have added additives and preservatives. Look for the list of ingredients to be the shortest possible e.g. 'Organic dried mango' as the single ingredient in one brand as opposed to 'Dried Mango, Preservative (Sodium Metabisulphite), added cane sugar' in another brand.

Trail mixes were originally made as combinations of snacks to be taken along on long hikes, but you can keep them in your car or take them to work where they will sit pretty on your desk. The nuts and seeds are full of heart-healthy fats and proteins and the dried fruit items are fibre dense. A handful of this is a very satisfying thing. If you like the sweet and savoury combination, you can add a dusting of paprika and a touch of salt to your trail mix.

1. Mix all the ingredients together and give them a good stir. Transfer into an airtight jar or large Tupperware box, making sure everything isn't packed together too tightly.

2. This will keep well for about 10 days.

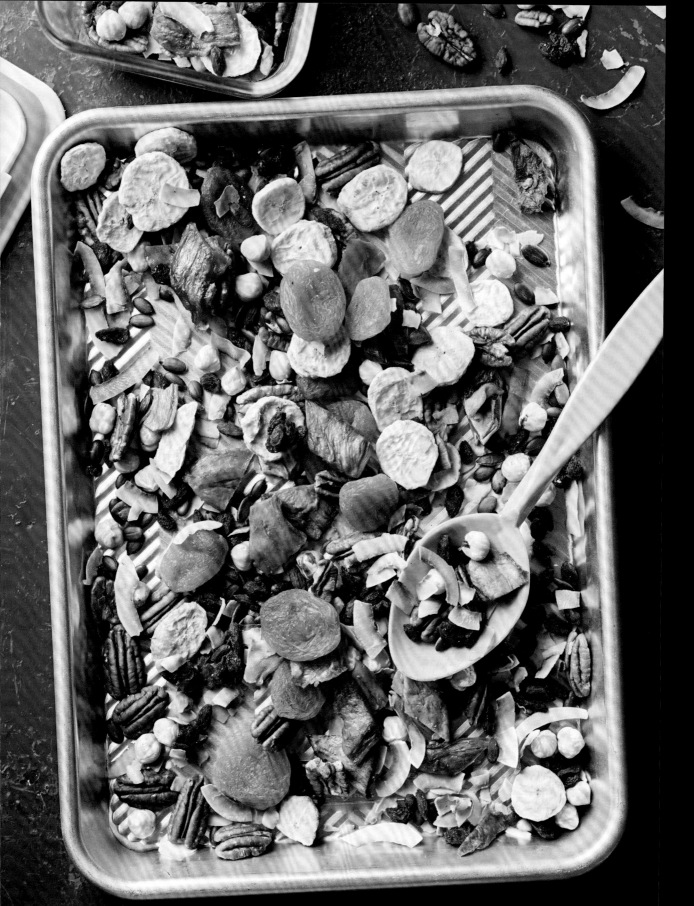

Sweet + Salty
Seaweed Crisps

MAKES 4 SERVINGS

Diversity points: 2 / Fibre: 1.4g

4 x 20cm (8in) square sheets of nori seaweed	
1–2 tbsp vegetable oil	
1 tsp sugar	
1 heaped teaspoon white sesame seeds	
Salt, to taste	

+ Bonus Diversity Points
Use a spice blend, for example shichimi togarashi, to add further spice diversity.

Crispy, umami, moreish – all the best elements of a snack. The sheets of nori seaweed I use are the same ones that are used to make sushi and can be found in the 'World Food' sections of most supermarkets. They are a rich source of the mineral iodine, which supports thyroid function.

1. Preheat the oven to 180°C fan/200°C/gas mark 6 and line a large baking tray with greaseproof paper.

2. Cut each nori sheet in half to form rectangles, and then into strips that are about 2cm (¾in) thick. This gives you pieces which look like long fingers. Place the seaweed on the lined baking tray, spreading them out evenly. Brush the nori sheets with the vegetable oil as evenly as you can, then sprinkle over the sugar and sesame seeds and season with salt to taste.

3. Bake in the oven for 6–8 minutes until the nori is crisp. Remove and allow to cool before serving. These will keep well in an airtight jar for a few days.

 Time Saving Hack
The fastest way of doing this is in the oven. The air fryer is not an option as the nori pieces fly up and attach themselves to the heated bars of the air fryer.

Snack Attack

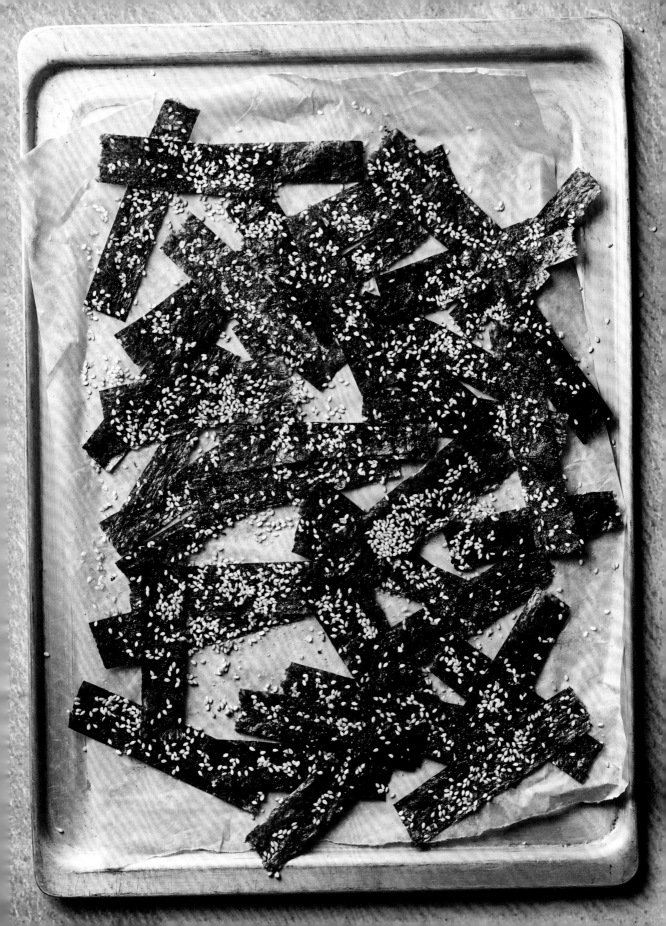

Chilli Lemon Crisps

Diversity points: 2 / Fibre: 2.7g

2 large flatbreads, about 30cm (12in) in diameter
1 tsp smoked paprika
½ tsp red chilli powder
2 generous tbsp extra-virgin olive oil
3 tbsp lemon juice
Salt, to taste

+ Bonus Diversity Points
The crisps themselves don't have a very high diversity score but you can up the score by serving them with an array of dips, like hummus or guacamole.

Here I use shop-bought flatbreads and my air fryer to make the crunchiest, most delicious crisps. The key is to look at the ingredients list and select a non-ultra-processed flatbread. I often go for either a lavash bread or the Crosta & Mollica brand.

1. Use scissors to cut your flatbreads into small triangles that resemble tortilla chips. Put the flatbread pieces into a large bowl and dust over the smoked paprika, red chilli powder, olive oil, lemon juice and salt. Mix gently so that all the pieces are coated evenly.

2. Transferred to the air fryer and spread them out evenly in the air fryer tray – you may need to do these in batches. Air fry at 180°C (325°F) for 6–8 minutes until they are golden and crisp; open the air fryer drawer and shake every couple of minutes or so to ensure even browning.

 Time Saving Hack
The fastest way of doing this recipe is in the air fryer but you can also use a conventional oven preheated to 180°C fan/200°C/gas mark 6 and bake these for about 10 minutes.

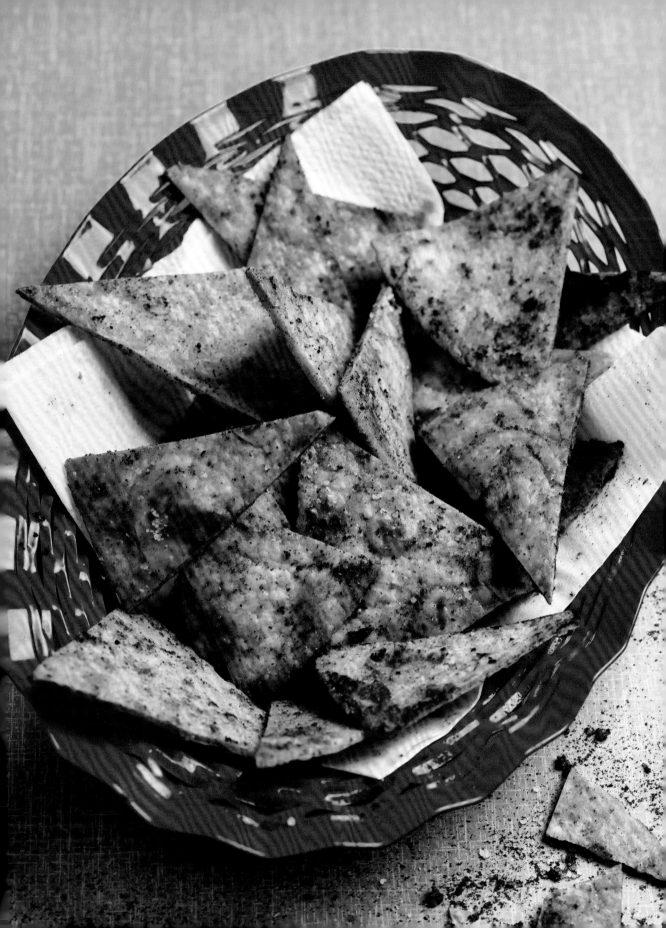

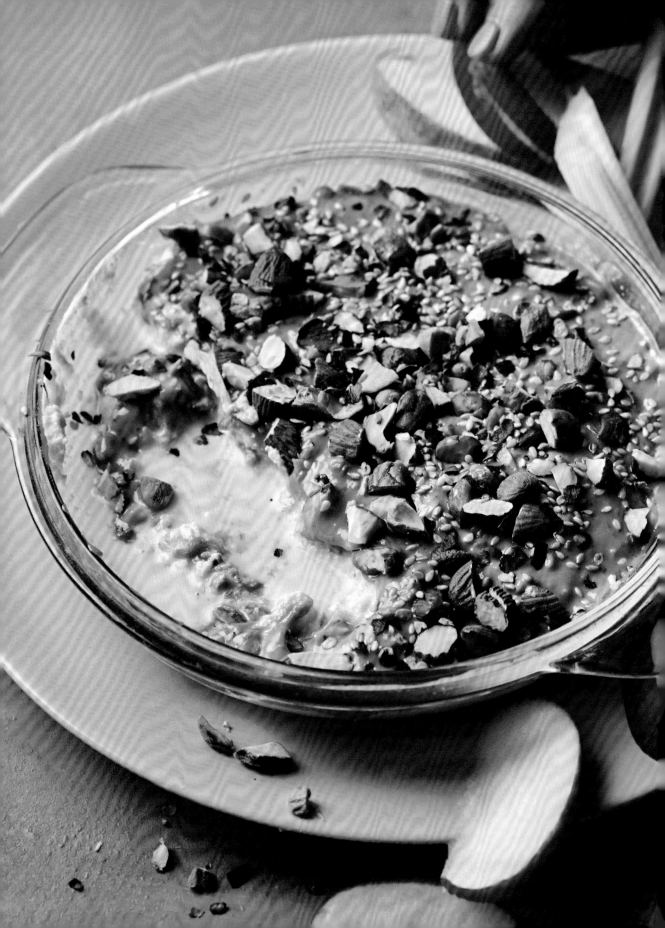

Ricotta + Nut Dip

Diversity points: 9 / Fibre: 5.6g

1 tsp honey or maple syrup

250g (9oz) mascarpone cheese

1 tbsp tahini

150g (5oz) crunchy peanut butter

1 tsp chilli flakes (optional)

2 tbsp plain almonds, roughly chopped

2 tbsp shelled pistachios, roughly chopped

1 tbsp sesame seeds

TO SERVE

1 apple, thinly sliced

4 celery sticks, cut into batons

2 large carrots, peeled and cut into batons

6 baby cucumbers, halved

1 head of chicory, leaves separated

+ Bonus Diversity Points
Add different nuts and seeds e.g. walnuts and cashew butter. Stud the mascarpone with dried figs and dates.

This is a delicious dip that you can prepare in advance and keep ready in your fridge. I serve it with slices of apple, celery and sometimes cucumber and carrots. It's particularly useful to feed to hungry children when they return from school and leftovers make a great toast topper.

1. Stir the honey into the mascarpone – I often do this straight into the tub the mascarpone comes in. Stir well to combine, then transfer to a shallow glass bowl.

2. Drizzle the tahini and peanut butter over the top, making sure that all the mascarpone is covered. Sprinkle over a few chilli flakes (if using) and scatter over the almonds and pistachios along with the sesame seeds. Chill in the fridge until ready to use. Serve with any or all of the fruits and vegetables listed.

Time Saving Hack
I use a nice runny peanut butter that is easy to drizzle over the mascarpone cheese. This saves me having to loosen, then spread the peanut butter with a knife. Look for bags of pre-prepared crudités in the supermarket if you are short on time.

Choco-Nut Popcorn Mix

Diversity points: 4 / Fibre: 4.8g

100g (3½oz) dark chocolate (at least 75% solids)
80g (7oz) salted popcorn from a packet (or homemade)
150g (5oz) toasted Brazil nuts
100g (3½oz) dried cranberries

+ Bonus Diversity Points
Add other nuts like walnuts or hazelnuts to your mix. You can also add toasted pumpkin or sunflower seeds.

A wonderfully balanced mixture of textures and flavours to have sitting in a jar in your living room. Popcorn is of course a popped whole grain, which makes it full of fibre, dark chocolate is an excellent source of gut-loving polyphenols and Brazil nuts are a particularly good source of the micronutrient selenium.

1. Roughly chop the dark chocolate into small pieces about the size of a 5p coin. Combine all the ingredients together in a bowl and mix well. Transfer to an airtight jar.

Time Saving Hack
I use popcorn from a packet to save time, but you can use the kernels to make your popcorn from scratch. Just add 2 tablespoons of popcorn seeds and 1 tablespoon of vegetable oil to a saucepan with a lid and place over a high heat. When the popcorn stops 'popping' remove from the heat and carefully remove the lid. The popcorn is ready!

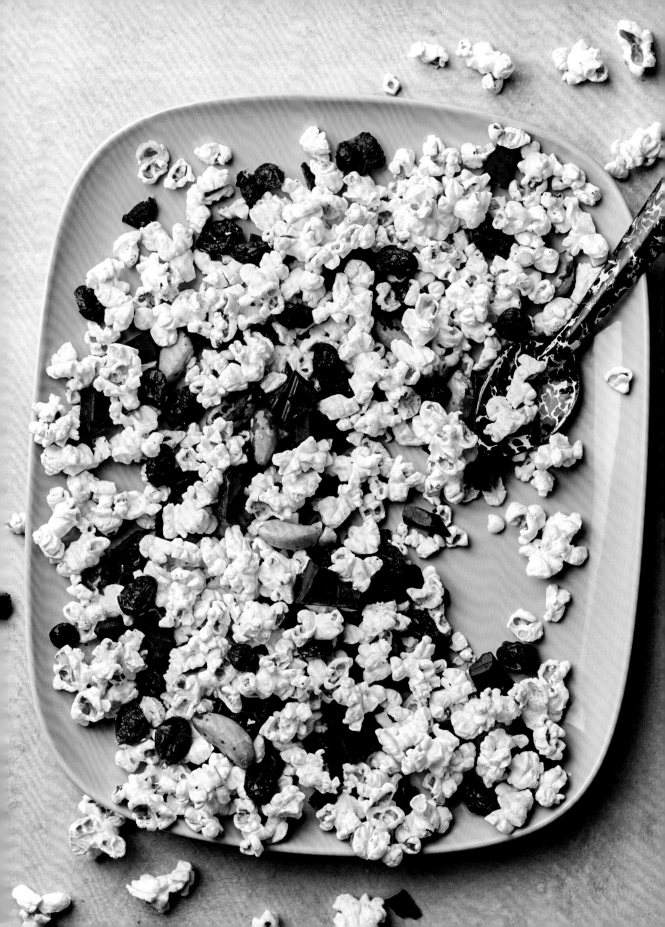

Coconut, Dark Chocolate, Ginger + Prune Clusters

Diversity points: 4 / Fibre: 6.1g (per cluster)

200g (7oz) dark chocolate (at least 75% cocoa solids) broken into pieces

100g (3½oz) desiccated coconut, plus 1 tablespoon for sprinkling

120g (4oz/½ cup) prunes, roughly chopped

100g (3½oz/⅔ cup) almonds, roughly chopped, plus a few to decorate

50g (2oz) stem ginger, roughly chopped

Sea salt crystals

1 tsp icing sugar (*optional*)

+ Bonus Diversity Points

Instead of almonds you can use a mixture of seeds e.g. pumpkin, sunflower or golden flaxseeds. Coffee is thought to contain a myriad of gut-friendly compounds so why not serve these cookies with a cup of espresso?

Time Saving Hack
You can use dark chocolate which has been flavoured with ginger or even orange if you prefer this to using stem ginger.

I guess you could consider this recipe the gut-healthy option for chocolate cookie lovers. Fibre-rich desiccated coconut is mixed with bitter dark chocolate, spiced ginger and sweet jammy prunes. Prunes are of course known to exert some laxative effect, making these cookies perfect for the constipated among us.

1. Start by melting the dark chocolate. I tend to do this in a bain marie (heatproof bowl placed over a saucepan of simmering water) as I have variable success in the microwave.

2. While the chocolate is melting, put the desiccated coconut into a small frying pan or saucepan and toast over a medium heat until it's golden brown. This will take 2–3 minutes and requires you to constantly stir so that the coconut does not catch.

3. Combine the desiccated coconut, prunes, almonds and stem ginger into the melted dark chocolate and mix well to combine.

4. Line a tray with some greaseproof paper. Spoon clusters of the mixture on to the tray and flatten gently with the back of the spoon. You're aiming to make around 10 cookies altogether. Sprinkle over a little extra desiccated coconut and chopped almonds for decoration, plus a few sea salt crystals.

5. Once the mixture has cooled slightly transfer to the fridge; as the mixture cools it will harden to form a firm cookie. If you wish, just before serving sprinkle over just a touch of icing sugar. It sticks to the irregular surfaces and make the cookies look very beautiful.

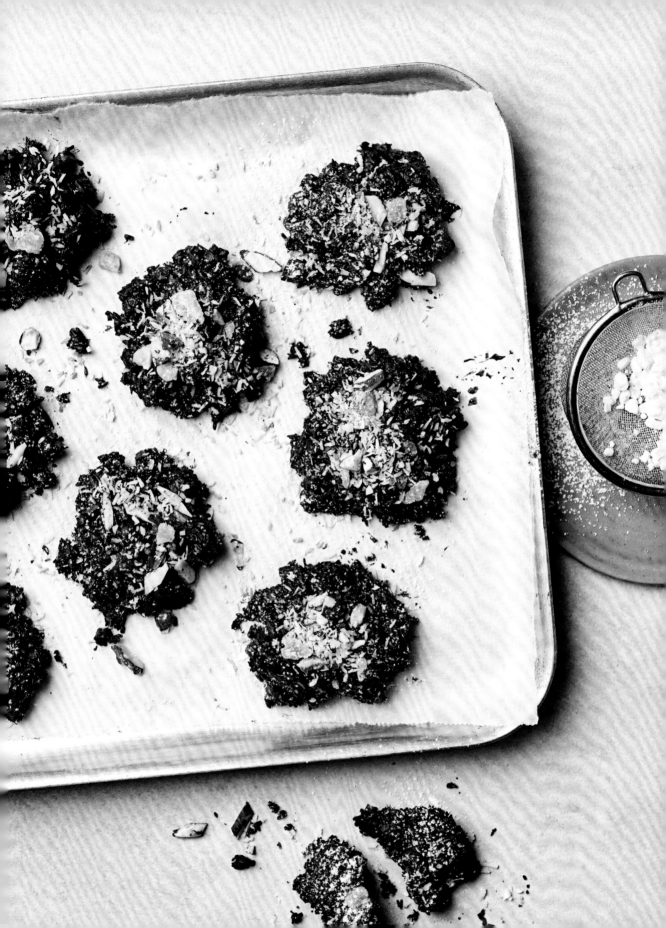

Spicy Mixed Seeds

Diversity points: 5 / Fibre: 4.1g (per serving)

200g (7oz) mixed seeds (pumpkin, sunflower and flaxseeds)

2 tsp granulated sugar

1 tbsp vegetable oil

1 heaped tsp harissa paste

½ tsp red chilli powder

½ tsp black pepper

Salt, to taste

+ Bonus Diversity Points
You can add nuts to this recipe e.g. pine nuts or almonds.

These are so crunchy, munchy and delicious – a tablespoon of this spicy seed mix and your taste buds will be left tingling. I use harissa paste with extra chilli powder and black pepper for full-on fire! This heat is tempered with a touch of sugar. The seeds also make a wonderful salad topper and keep well in a jar for a few weeks.

1. Place a non-stick frying pan over a medium heat. Add the mixed seeds, a teaspoon of the sugar and the vegetable oil to the frying pan and stir well to combine. Allow the seeds to toast for around a minute or two before adding the harissa, chilli powder and black pepper. Make sure you continue to stir the seeds so they don't catch.

2. When the seeds start turning a golden colour add another teaspoon of sugar and season with salt. Stir well to combine. After a minute or so, tip the seeds out onto a tray lined with greaseproof paper and spread them out so that they have space to cool.

3. Store the seeds in an airtight jar to keep them crunchy.

 Time Saving Hack
Instead of spending time weighing out three different types of seed, I just buy a bag of mixed seeds. The different seed varieties all have different colours and textures, so they do look quite special together.

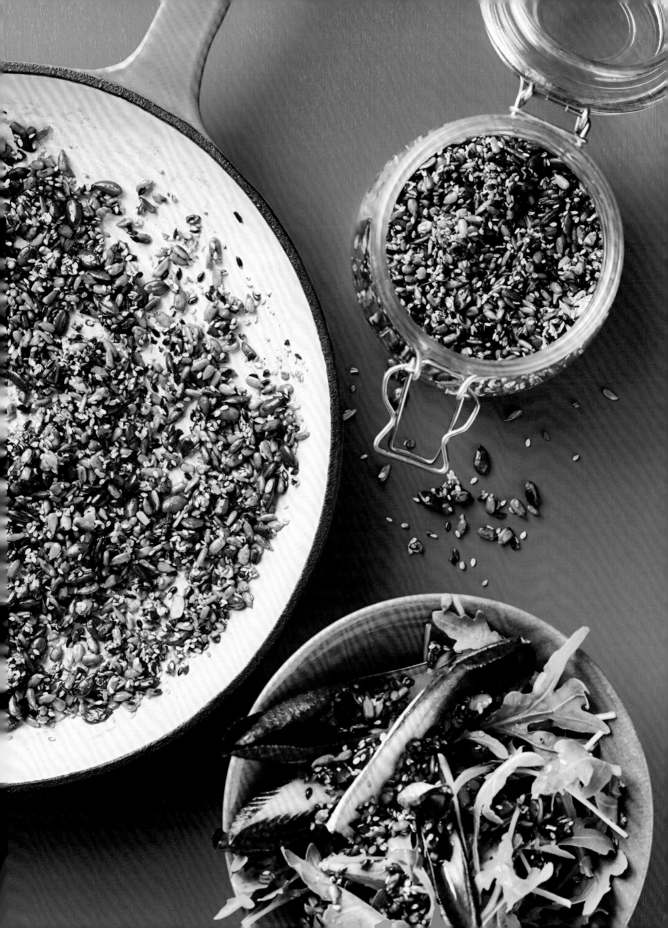

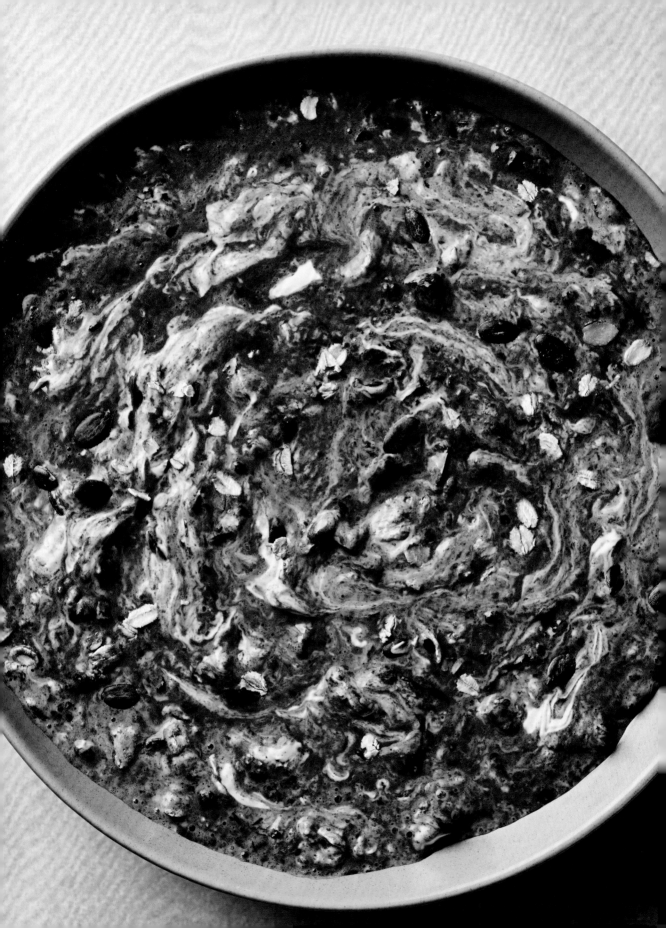

Cherry, Blackberry + Rose Yoghurt

Diversity points: 4 / Fibre: 1.9g

200g (7oz) frozen sour pitted Morello cherries

200g (7oz) frozen blackberries

2 tbsp maple syrup

1 tsp rosewater

500g (1lb 2oz) full-fat live Greek yoghurt

1–2 tbsp jumbo oats

1 tbsp pumpkin seeds

+ Bonus Diversity Points

Add any mixture of frozen berries that you have available. Strawberries and blueberries are wonderful, as are pre-prepared frozen summer fruit mixes.

I became so fed up with those supposedly 'healthy', low-fat flavoured yoghurts that are in fact full of additives, emulsifiers and preservatives that I decided to make my own at home. I have never looked back. This recipe is infinitely superior in my opinion to anything else on the market. Give it a try and you will know what I mean. The rosewater really is optional, but the very distant floral tone just enhances the flavour of the berries.

1. Start by putting your sour cherries and blackberries into a large bowl and drizzling over the maple syrup. Transfer to the microwave for 2 minutes, then use a potato masher to gently mash the fruit into a rough purée-like consistency.

2. Allow the fruit mixture to cool for a couple of minutes, then add the rosewater, yoghurt, oats and pumpkin seeds and stir well. Refrigerate until you're ready to serve – it will thicken slightly as it cools.

Time Saving Hack
You can just add the cherries and blackberries from frozen straight into the yoghurt but be aware that they do release a little liquid so you'll need to stir the yoghurt well before serving.

Seafood Dips with Crackers

Two dip recipes that you are bound to fall in love with. The first uses smoked salmon and is perfect to have ready in the fridge for when you want something a little premium to snack on. The second uses canned tuna and an unexpected addition, lime pickle! This really brings out the tuna's 'A game'. I serve with sourdough crackers, or any other artisan variety of cracker (the browner and seedier the better). Try to find a cracker variety that doesn't contain a million additives or preservatives and has a relatively high fibre content.

+ Bonus Diversity Points
Serve with extra crudités such as cucumbers, carrots, radishes and even endive or radicchio.

Time Saving Hack
Make the dips ahead of time, so that they are ready for when the urge to snack strikes. The mixtures keep well in the fridge for up to 3 days.

Lemony Salmon + Herb Dip
Diversity points: 4 / Fibre: 7.1g

100g (3½oz) smoked salmon

½ x 400g (12oz) can butter beans (120g/4oz drained weight)

120g (4oz) cream cheese

Juice of 1 lemon

Handful of dill, plus a little extra to garnish

1 spring onion, roughly chopped

Extra-virgin olive oil, for drizzling

Crackers, to serve

1. Start by placing the smoked salmon, beans, cream cheese and lemon juice into a food processor and blitzing to a coarse purée.

2. Add the dill and spring onion and blitz again until the spring onion has broken down. Spoon the mixture into a deep bowl. Drizzle over a little extra-virgin olive oil and scatter over the dill before serving with crackers.

Whipped Tuna + Lime Pickle Dip
Diversity points: 2 / Fibre: 4.6g

2 x 145g (5oz) tins tuna in spring water, drained

2 tsp lime pickle, plus a little extra for drizzling

Juice of 1 lemon

150g (5oz) cottage cheese

100g (3½oz) cream cheese

¼ red onion, roughly chopped, plus a little extra to garnish

Handful of coriander

1. Place the drained tuna, the lime pickle, lemon juice, cottage cheese and cream cheese in a food processor and blitz until it forms a smooth purée. Add the red onion and the coriander and blitz again until the onion has broken down into the tuna mixture.

2. Spoon the mixture into a deep bowl. Drizzle over a little extra lime pickle and scatter the red onion.

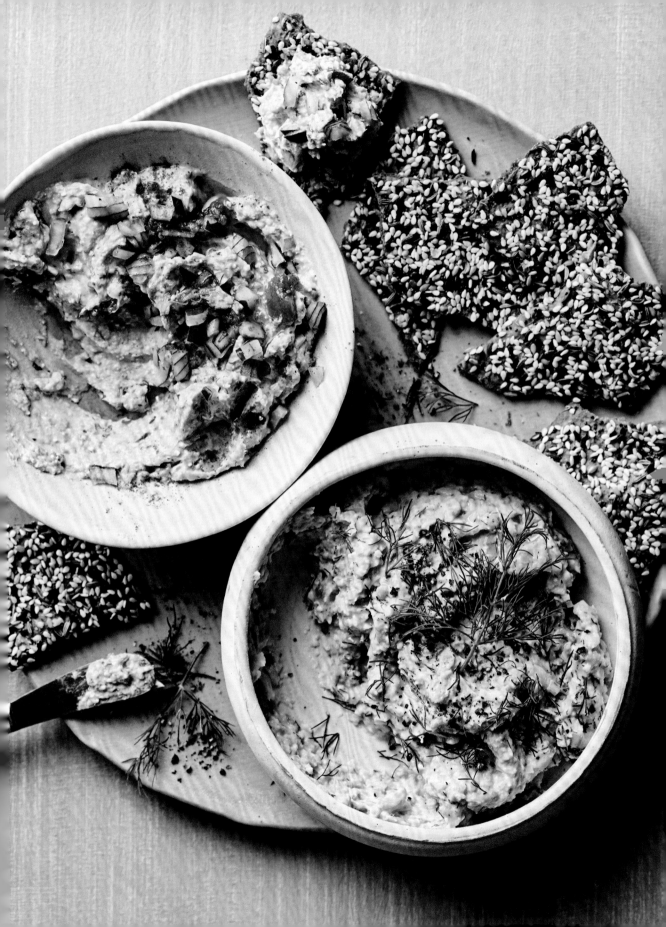

Bliss Balls

Diversity points: 8 / Fibre: 3.3g

200g (7oz) packet of fruit, nut and seed mix

2 tbsp jumbo rolled oats

½ tsp ground cinnamon

½–1 tsp fennel seeds

½ tsp nigella seeds

2 cardamom pods, bashed to release the seeds

8 juicy Medjool dates, pitted

75g (2¾oz) white and/or black sesame seeds

+ Bonus Diversity Points

For a chocolatey alternative why not add cacao powder to the mix? Matcha lovers can add matcha powder instead of the spices I have listed.

'Bliss balls' are often considered a healthy snack alternative because they contain naturally occurring sugars rather than added processed, refined sugars. They are by no means 'sugar-free' but do contain plenty of nuts, seeds and spices for extra diversity. Perfect as a pre-workout snack, an after-dinner sweet treat or even as a quick pick-me-up in the morning for breakfast.

1. Place the fruit, nut and seed mix, oats, cinnamon, fennel seeds, nigella seeds and cardamom seeds into a food processor. Blitz for a minute or two until the mixture is really fine.

2. Add the dates to the food processor along with 1–2 tablespoons of kettle-hot water. Blitz again – the mixture should start coming together and forming a cohesive lump in the food processor as you blitz it. At this point, when it has all come together, stop blitzing any further.

3. Take rough tablespoons of the mixture in the palms of your hand and roll into walnut-sized balls. Oiling your hands slightly can make it easier to shape the mixture into balls.

4. Tip the sesame seeds on to a plate, then roll the bliss balls in the sesame seeds until they are coated all over. Store in a single layer in a Tupperware container in the fridge.

Time Saving Hack
You save time measuring out individual ingredients by buying a packet of mixed fruit, nuts and seeds that already weighs 200g (7oz).

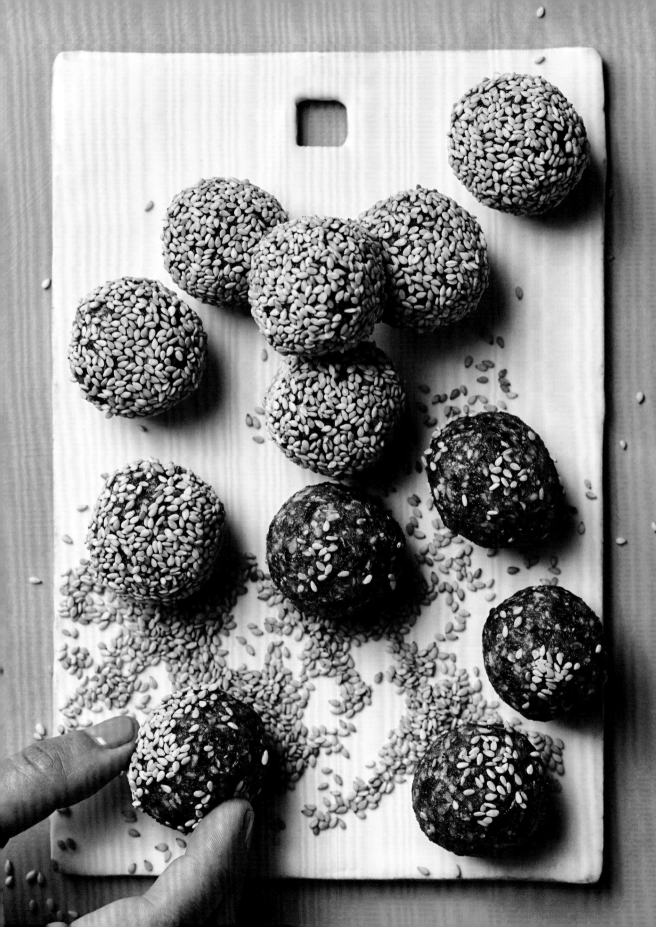

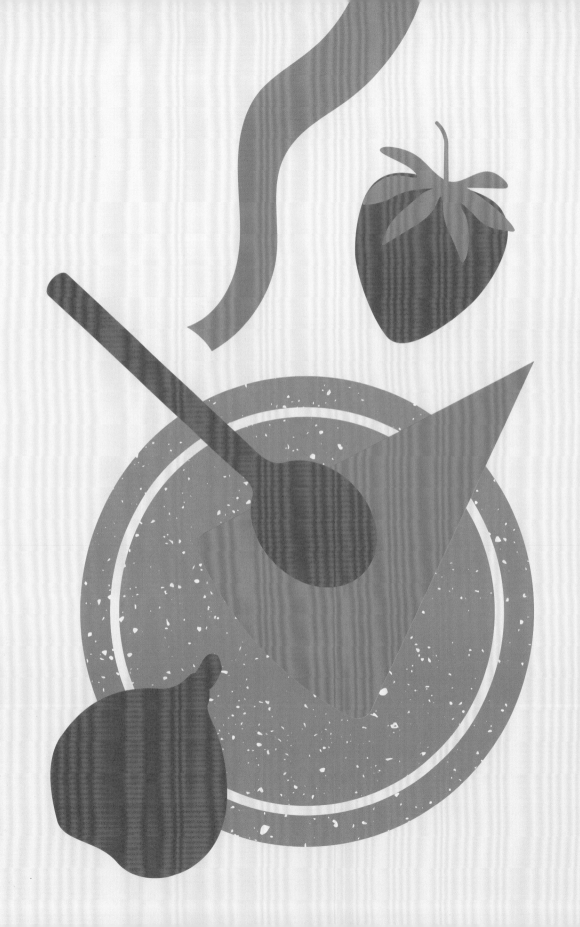

Speedy Sweet Treats

It is nearly impossible to envisage modern life without sugar. We celebrate our birthdays, weddings and anniversaries with cake, we finish our fancy meals with a sweet pudding – even breastmilk is sweet. We bribe our kids (and ourselves) with sweets and chocolates because our bodies and brains respond immediately to sugar, hard-wired as they are to seek out the fastest source of energy.

But what is so special about sugar? Why, when we are full to bursting after a massive feast, do our bodies suddenly find extra space when someone mentions dessert? What is this sorcery that can create additional stomach space where none existed before?

The answer lies in what our bodies have evolved to do. Early in the human journey, when energy sources may have been in short supply, it was vital that we were able to ingest any and all sources of energy, especially energy-dense sugars like ripe fruit. And being full was no excuse! When we didn't know where or when the next meal would be, it was vital that nothing was left to waste.

Nowadays, supermarkets exist, and our lifestyles are more 'sit at a desk' than 'wrestle a sabre-toothed tiger for the next meal', and as a result our hunting and gathering skills have been repurposed. But that evolutionary trait still exists, telling our brains to eat that packet of Jammie Dodgers just in case we need to outrun a woolly mammoth sometime this afternoon.

But aside from the evolutionary aspect of sugar consumption, there is also the concept of 'hedonic' hunger signals, which govern how much sweet food we consume. This is a fancy way of saying that we eat sweet foods because sugar triggers our brain's reward centres, releasing feel-good chemicals like dopamine, serotonin and endorphins. These make us feel happy.

But that happiness quickly gives way to a plethora of less positive consequences. For example, eating too much sugar has a massive impact on gut health. Lots of sweet food can cause an abundance of species like Proteobacteria and a simultaneous decrease in Bacteroidetes, which can lead to a potential weakening of the gut's barrier function and even cause a degree of inflammation in the gut.

So, sugar triggers our feel-good chemicals, and we are evolutionarily hard-wired to find it and eat it. But it also is pretty bad for our gut and digestion, not to mention what it can do to our teeth. So, what's the answer? What can we do in the face of such pressure?

First and foremost, try to reduce the number of sugary ultra-processed food items you buy. Studies suggest that by reducing ultra-processed food consumption you can roughly halve the number of free sugars in your diet. This is where the delicious desserts in this chapter come in (as well as some of the sweet items in the snack chapter). These recipes have been designed so that they contain a huge number of other beneficial items such as polyphenol-rich chocolate, nutrient-rich fruits, and the live probiotic goodness of yoghurt and kefir.

Moderation is, of course, key, and there is no better advice that I can give when it comes to reining in the sweet tooth. We all exist somewhere along a continuum with sugar: some of us will do anything for that sugar and dopamine rush, while others are less fussed. The same person can switch from one state to the other over the course of a lifetime. So, it's worth taking a moment to reflect on where you feel you lie on the sugar continuum before deciding on the right strategy for lowering your sugar intake.

Earl Grey + Dark Chocolate Mousse

Diversity points: 2 / Fibre: 4.1g

200g (7oz) dark chocolate (at least 70% cocoa solids)
200ml (7fl oz/generous ¾ cup) kettle-hot water
3–4 Earl Grey teabags
Good-quality extra-virgin olive oil, for drizzling
Maldon sea salt flakes
Drizzle of tahini and a few toasted pine nuts (optional)

+ Bonus Diversity Points
Add a selection of toasted and finely chopped nuts to the mousse. Flavour the tea with fennel and cardamom or even cinnamon and cloves.

Time Saving Hack
I'm afraid I have no method of making chocolate set rapidly, but the beauty of this dish is that it takes just 10–12 minutes to prepare, so it can easily be made in advance.

Considering this contains so few ingredients, it's deeply satisfying. Using 70% dark chocolate with a high cocoa content is a must, as are good-quality Earl Grey teabags. Both dark chocolate and tea are rich sources of polyphenols, plant compounds that can be beneficial for our gut bugs. The mousse is quite rich, so you really don't need much. If you are handy with a metal spoon, serving the mousse in quenelles looks impressive.

1. Put the kettle on to boil. Pour some boiling water into a saucepan and place over a low heat, then sit a heatproof bowl over the pan, making sure the base of the bowl doesn't touch the water. Break the chocolate into small pieces and add them to the bowl, stirring gently until they melt.

2. While the chocolate is melting, put the teabags into a measuring jug and pour in the kettle-hot water. Stir gently to brew the tea.

3. When the chocolate has melted, remove it from the heat. Remove the teabags from the brewed tea. Slowly pour the tea into the melted chocolate, stirring really well - the mixture might seem to seize up initially, but continuous stirring will bring it back to a smooth consistency like a chocolate sauce or soup. Pour the mixture into a bowl or individual ramekins and transfer to the fridge. Chill for at least 4–6 hours, but ideally overnight to allow the mousse to set.

4. Use a metal spoon soaked in hot water to make quenelles of the mousse but don't worry about making them perfect. Serve the mousse topped with a drizzle of olive oil and some sea salt. If you like you can also drizzle over a tiny amount of tahini and some toasted pine nuts.

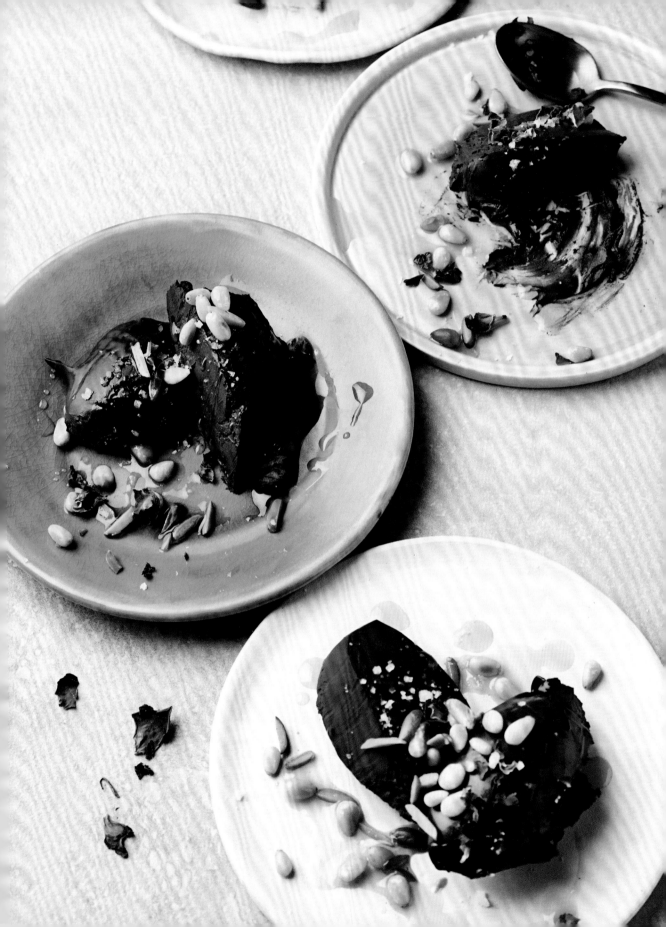

Caramelised Plantains with Sesame

Diversity points: 3 / Fibre: 5.1g

2 large ripe plantains

2 tbsp vegetable oil

½ tsp ground cinnamon

¼ tsp grated nutmeg

2 heaped tbsp soft light brown sugar

2 tbsp white sesame seeds

Salt, to taste

200g (7oz) soured cream/crème fraîche/Greek yoghurt, to serve

+ Bonus Diversity Points
Add toasted mixed nuts or seeds to the caramelised plantains before serving.

Plantains are naturally higher in fibre than bananas and are rich in vitamins A and C, as well as potassium and magnesium. They are ideal for use in both savoury and sweet dishes, but really do come to life here in this caramelised plantain dish. For best results try and pick a plantain that is not too unripe.

1. Start by peeling the plantains and cutting them into approximately 1.5cm (½in) thick coins.

2. Heat a large non-stick frying pan over a low-medium heat. Drizzle in the oil and place the plantains in the frying pan. Try not to overload the pan, you need to keep the plantains in a single layer. If the frying pan is looking too full, spread the plantains across two frying pans.

3. Fry the plantains for 3–4 minutes on one side, until they start turning a deep golden colour and are slightly softened. Turn the plantains over and fry the other side for about 2 minutes before dusting over the cinnamon, nutmeg and sugar. The sugar will start to melt and turn into a caramel almost immediately. Stir the caramel into the plantains and when all the plantains are coated, scatter over the sesame seeds. Remove the plantains from the pan, season with a touch of salt and serve immediately with cool soured cream, crème fraîche or yoghurt.

 Time Saving Hack
Using a slightly riper plantain and slicing it thinly speeds up the cooking time significantly.

Speedy Sweet Treats

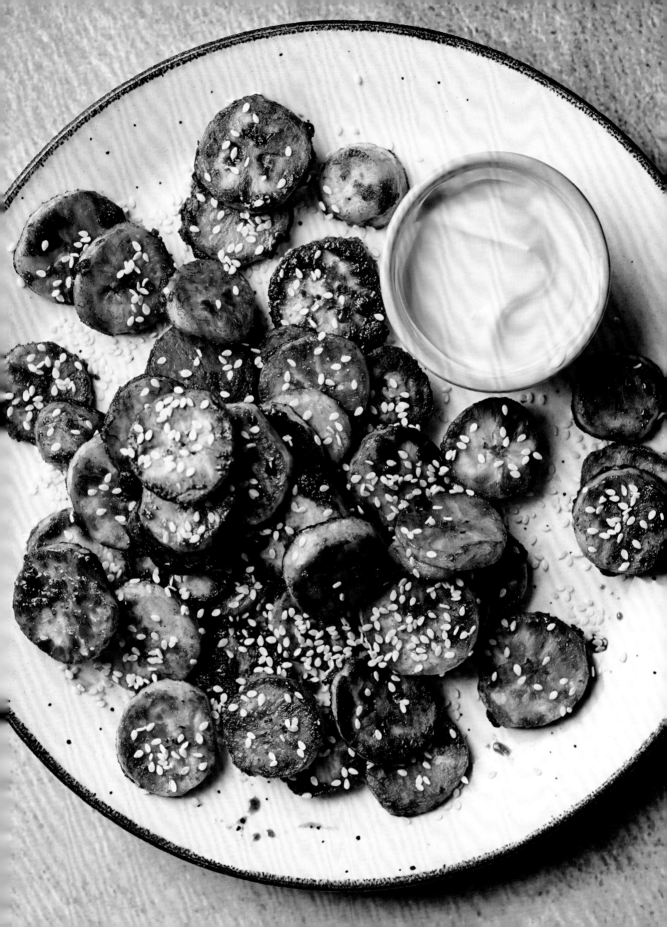

Ras el Hanout Poached Pears + Peaches

Diversity points: 6 / Fibre: 4.2g

3 tbsp soft light brown sugar

1 x 410g (14oz) tin peach halves in juice

1 x 410g (14oz) tin pear halves in juice

1 tsp ras el hanout spice mix

Pinch of saffron

2 tbsp toasted pistachios, roughly chopped

2 tbsp toasted almonds, roughly chopped

2 tbsp toasted hazelnuts, roughly chopped

Salt, to taste

+ Bonus Diversity Points
Serve the fruit with overnight oats or even granola.

A cheat's dish if there ever was one. Tinned pears and peaches are gently warmed through in a spiced syrup and scattered with toasted nuts. It gives the illusion that you have spent hours slow-poaching the fruit yourself, and the texture is just delightful. Leftovers make a fantastic breakfast the next day with kefir yoghurt and granola.

1. Tip the sugar into a wide saucepan and place over a medium heat. After about 2 minutes you'll see the sugar starting to caramelise; at this point pour in about two-thirds of the juice from one of the tins of fruit. The sugar will immediately turn solid but don't panic, in just a minute or two it will dissolve again. Keep stirring the sugar and the juice until it starts to reduce and thicken. Add the ras el hanout and saffron to the syrup and stir well to combine. You are looking for something with the consistency of maple syrup.

2. Drain the rest of the fruit in a colander and discard (or drink!) the juice. Gently add the drained fruit to the syrup and use a spoon to 'baste' the fruit with the spiced syrup. Simmer for just a minute or two to warm the fruit through.

3. Pour the fruit into a large, deep bowl. Scatter the chopped nuts over the fruit and season with just a touch of salt to break the sweetness. Serve warm or cold.

 Time Saving Hack
Using a spice mix like ras el hanout or baharat is quicker than having to measure out individual spices. Tinned fruit is already poached, so it saves you the effort of slow-poaching yourself. Food sorcery at its best.

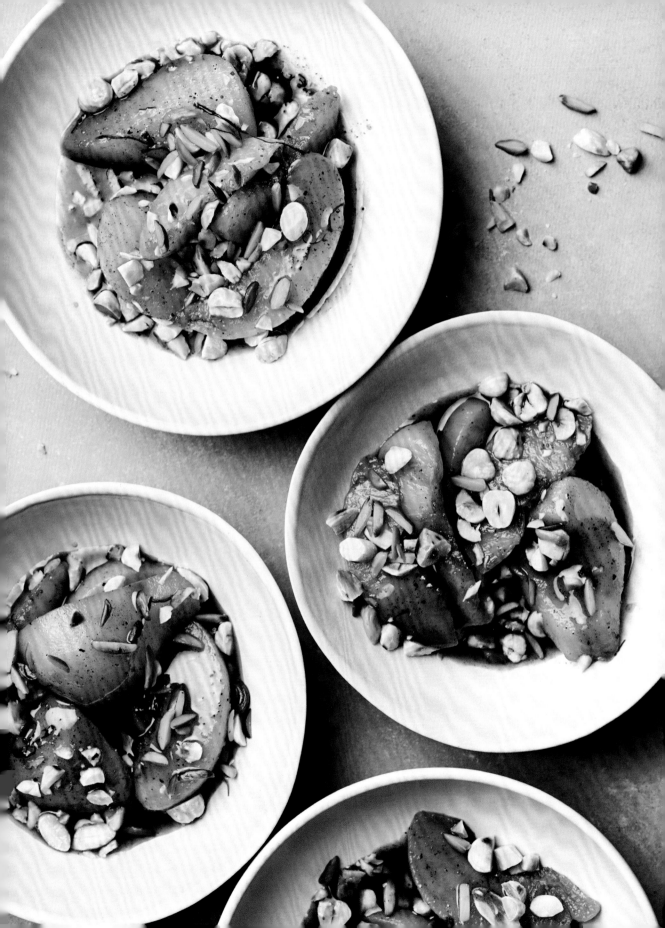

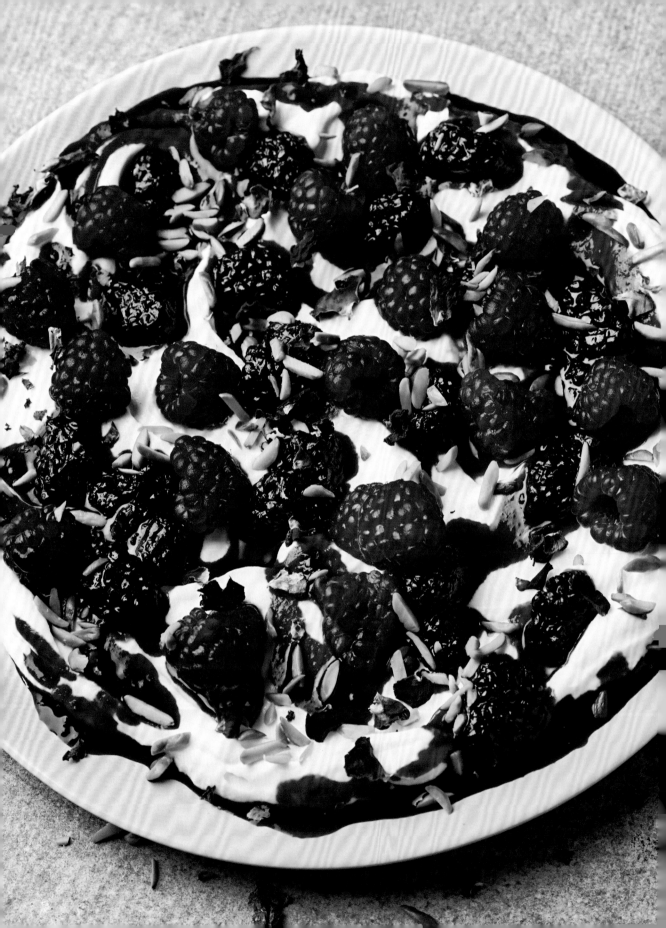

Labneh with Swirled Berries + Elderflower

Diversity points: 3 / Fibre: 3.8g

350g (12oz) labneh (or full-fat live Greek yoghurt)
4 tbsp elderflower cordial
1 tbsp soft light brown sugar
200g (7oz) blackberries
Seeds of 1 cardamom pod
100g (3½oz) raspberries
50g (2oz) slivered pistachios
Dried rose petals (optional)

+ Bonus Diversity Points

Mango, pineapple and passionfruit would also work well, perhaps with toasted coconut flakes. For a protein boost replace the labneh with Skyr, a high-protein yoghurt from Iceland.

Labneh is a strained yoghurt now available online and in certain supermarkets. You can make your own by hanging Greek yoghurt overnight in a muslin cloth (making sure you have a bowl underneath to catch the whey). Organic elderflower cordial is a delicious way of imparting a gentle, summery flavour and complements the berries beautifully.

1. Mix the labneh with 3 tablespoons of the cordial and stir well to combine, then spread the elderflower labneh over a platter.

2. Put the brown sugar, half the blackberries and cardamom seeds in a saucepan and place over a medium heat. Use the back of a spoon to break the blackberries down slightly and cook for about 3 minutes, or until they are thick and jammy. Add the rest of the blackberries and stir through, then remove from the heat and allow to cool slightly before adding the remaining tablespoon of cordial.

3. Spoon the blackberries over the labneh as artistically as you can. Scatter over the fresh raspberries, pistachios and rose petals (if using). Serve immediately.

 Time Saving Hack

If you don't have time to cook your fruit, just macerate very ripe berries with icing sugar instead of soft brown sugar and smash them gently with a fork before layering on to the yoghurt.

Gut-Loving
Fig Pudding

Diversity points: 3 / Fibre: 4.9g

200g (7oz) soft dried figs
250ml (13fl oz / 1½ cups) whole milk
175g (6oz) full-fat live Greek yoghurt
Salt, to taste

OPTIONAL TOPPINGS

4 tbsp pomegranate seeds
Toasted flaked almonds
4 sliced fresh figs

+ Bonus Diversity Points

Add spices like cinnamon, nutmeg, fennel and cardamom to the milk before blitzing. You can add other dried fruit like prunes, dates or apricots.

Based on a classic Turkish recipe, this pudding is sweet and silky, almost like a fig custard. The magic is that it only contains three ingredients: fibre-dense dried figs, milk and yoghurt. You can add warm, earthy spices like cinnamon if you wish, but I like the natural flavour of the figs to come through.

1. Place the figs in a measuring jug and top up the jug with milk until it reaches the 375ml (13fl oz) mark. Place the measuring jug in the microwave for 2½ minutes, watching carefully to make sure that the milk doesn't boil over.

2. Pour the fig and milk mixture into a blender and blitz to a smooth purée. Add the yoghurt and a pinch of salt and give the mixture one further quick blitz to combine well. Transfer the fig mixture into either individual ramekins or one large bowl. You can serve this either straight away or allow it to cool before chilling in the fridge.

3. Serve with your pomegranate seeds, toasted flaked almonds and/or sliced fresh figs, if you like.

Time Saving Hack
The blender really does all the hard work here, so you don't have to.

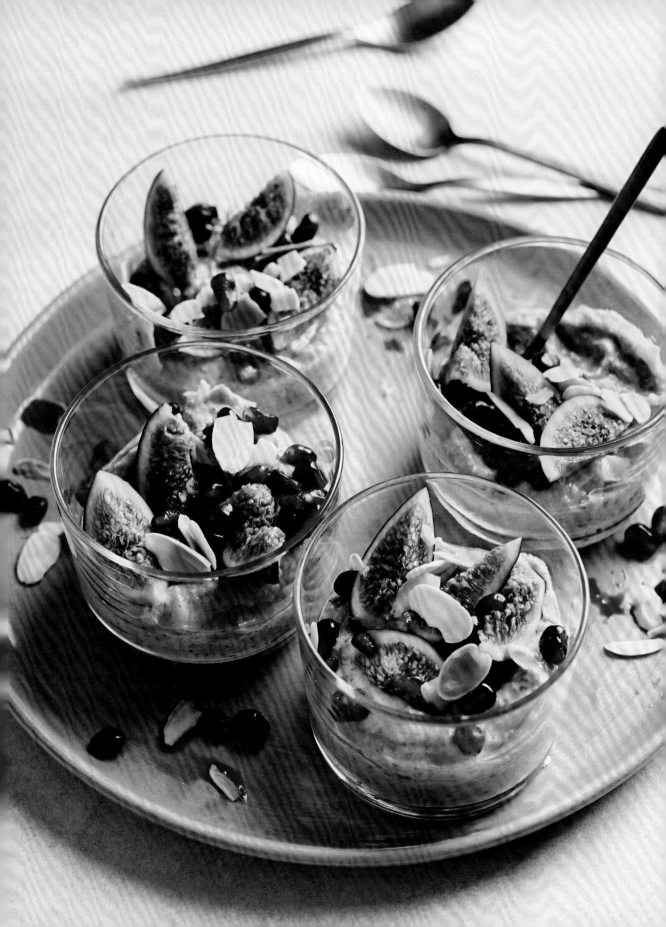

Iced Tutti
Frutti Parfait

Diversity points: 4 / Fibre: 6.9g

200g (7oz) frozen strawberries, semi-defrosted

2 generous tbsp maple syrup

2 kiwi fruit, peeled and cut into bite-sized chunks

150g (5oz) tinned pineapple chunks (in juice)

1 heaped tsp chia seeds

Juice of 1 lime

2 tsp rosewater (optional)

6 tbsp finely crushed ice/shaved

300g (10oz) soured cream or kefir yoghurt

+ Bonus Diversity Points

Use any frozen berry or combination of berries instead of strawberries if you wish. You can use frozen Morello cherries or even other fruit like from mango and pineapple. Tinned fruit would also work well here instead of frozen fruit.

I tried an outstanding version of this dessert in a roadside restaurant in Dubai so just had to try and make a gut-friendly version. The strawberries have a really syrupy texture. The trick is to use frozen strawberries (fresh strawberries don't grow in Dubai) and smash them; they release their sticky, saucy juices and make for the most delicious of fruity desserts.

1. Put the strawberries into a bowl with the maple syrup, then use a potato masher to give the fruit and syrup a good smash; it will start releasing its syrupy juice.

2. Add the kiwi fruit and pineapple to the strawberry syrup along with the chia seeds, lime juice and rosewater. Give the mixture a good smash with the masher to break the fruit down a little and help it release some of its juices.

3. To assemble the parfait, layer the crushed fruit with the ice in two individual glass bowls and top each with a tablespoon of soured cream or yoghurt. Repeat the process twice more to create three layers of iced fruit and cream. Serve immediately before the ice melts.

 ## Time Saving Hack
Prepare the fruit sauce in advance and have ready in the fridge – just layer up with the ice and soured cream when you are ready to serve the dessert.

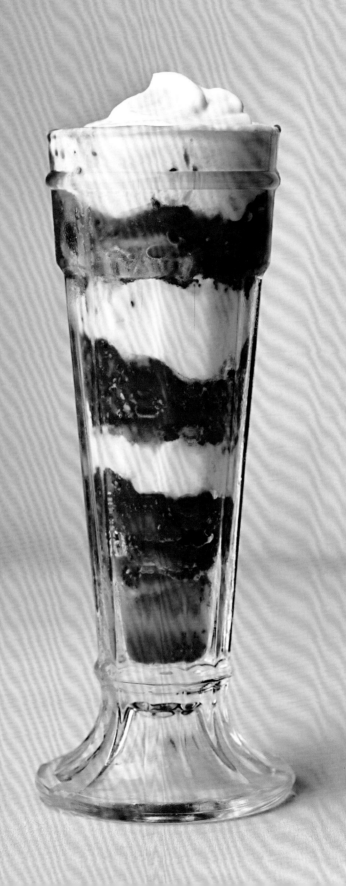

Pick + Mix Cheesecake

Diversity points: 8 / Fibre: 7.1g

90g (3¼oz) sourdough crackers (I like Peter's Yard Fig and Spelt Sourdough Crackers)

350g (12oz) mascarpone

1 heaped tbsp honey

1 heaped tsp vanilla bean paste

50g (2oz) raspberries

50g (2oz) strawberries

50g (2oz) blueberries

50g (2oz) mango chunks

50g (2oz) pineapple chunks

50g (2oz) ripe peaches (or use tinned peaches)

100g (3½oz) toasted pistachios

100g (3½oz) roasted hazelnuts

+ Bonus Diversity Points
Add toasted pumpkin seeds, almonds and flaxseeds to the platter. Or try chunks of banana and dark chocolate curls.

This is more of a guideline than a recipe. Start with a biscuit base (a crunchy sourdough cracker) and top with sweetened mascarpone, fruit and nuts. Children will enjoy this dessert and it works well at parties and picnics too.

1. Start by arranging the crackers on one side of a large platter.

2. Tip the mascarpone into a bowl, add the honey and vanilla paste and beat together until combined. Place the bowl on the platter.

3. Prepare all the fruit, cutting any larger fruit into small chunks, and arrange artistically on the platter. Roughly chop the nuts and arrange them on the platter as well.

4. Make your own combination of cheesecake by spooning the cheesecake filling on to the crackers and then topping with fruit and nuts of your choice.

Time Saving Hack
There is no time spent waiting for the cheesecake filling to set in this recipe, you only need a few minutes to chop up fruit and whip up the mascarpone.

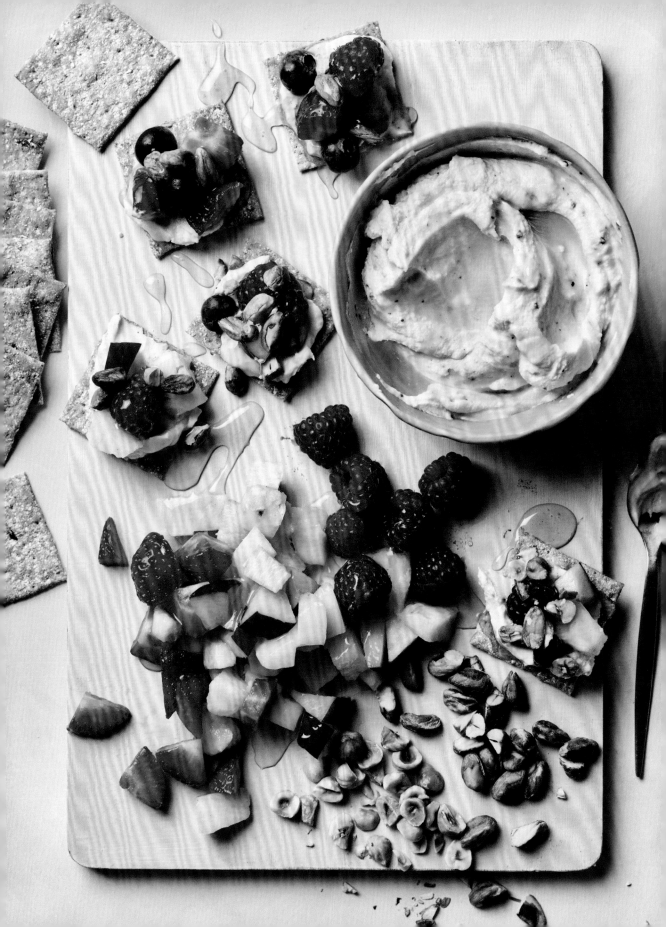

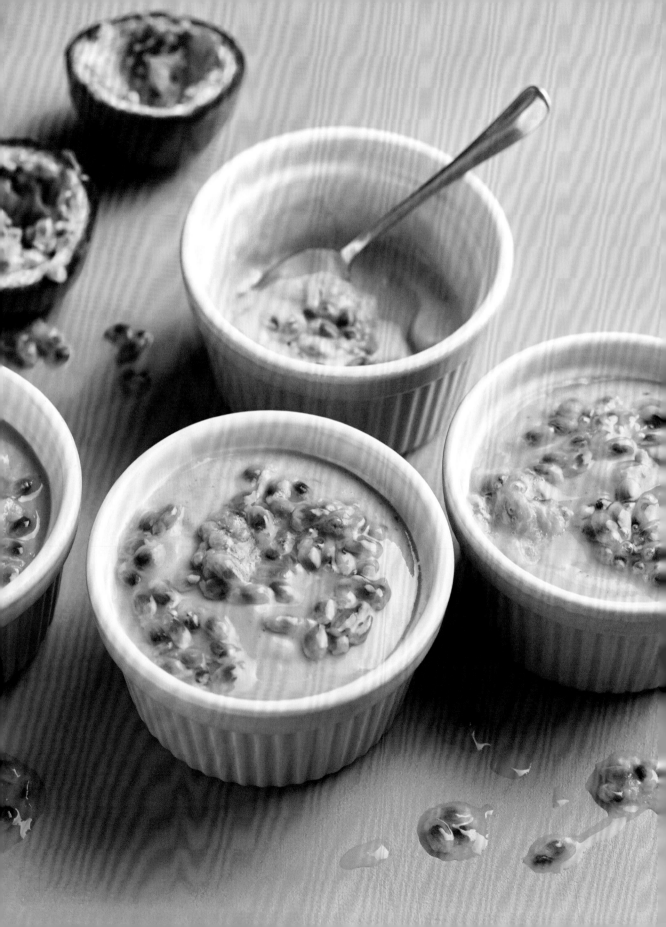

Mango + Passion Fruit Custard

Diversity points: 4 / Fibre: 1.7g

300g (10oz) silken tofu
3 tbsp lemon juice
200ml (7fl oz/generous ¾ cup) tinned alphonso mango pulp
1 medium ripe banana
2 tsp rosewater
Seeds of 2–3 cardamom pods
2 large passion fruit, halved

+ Bonus Diversity Points
Top the custard with chopped pistachios and extra chunks of fresh mango.

A block of silken tofu is used to make this perfectly smooth, wibbly-wobbly custard. A tin of alphonso mango pulp is used to sweeten and perfume the dish while banana gives it a thick, creamy texture. Do make sure you blend thoroughly to combine all the ingredients well, there must be no lumps.

1. Put all the ingredients except the passion fruit into a blender and blitz to a really smooth purée. Pour the mixture out into individual glasses or ramekins.

2. Scoop the passion fruit seeds and juice over the custard and eat immediately, or refrigerate and top with the passion fruit just before serving.

Time Saving Hack
Using tinned mango pulp means that you don't need to spend ages peeling, deseeding and then blending the mango to a purée yourself. You can freeze any leftover tinned mango pulp in ice lolly moulds to make wonderfully fruity ice lollies.

Charred Pineapple with Ginger + Black Pepper Syrup

Diversity points: 3 / Fibre: 2.9g

1 medium fresh pineapple

2 thumb-sized pieces of fresh ginger, julienned

3 tbsp maple syrup

½ tsp ground turmeric

½ tsp coarse black pepper

50g (2oz) butter

Frozen yoghurt, to serve (*optional*)

+ Bonus Diversity Points
Top the pineapple with toasted coconut and serve with live yoghurt spiked with lime juice and zest.

Tropical pineapple, charred to perfection and bursting with sweet, caramelised juice, is paired with spicy black pepper and ginger to create a marriage made in dessert heaven. This is particularly good with a good-quality shop-bought frozen yoghurt.

1. Top and tail the pineapple, then place it upright on your work surface. Cut away the outer peel of the pineapple and then slice it lengthways into quarters and remove the central core. Cut each pineapple quarter in half lengthways, so that you have a total of 8 pieces.

2. Place the ginger, maple syrup, turmeric and black pepper into a small saucepan with 3–4 tablespoons of water. Bring the mixture to the boil, then lower the heat and simmer for about 5 minutes to reduce down into a spiced syrup.

3. Meanwhile, place a large non-stick frying pan over a medium-high heat. Add half the butter to the pan and when it is bubbling, add half the pineapple. Cook the pineapple in the butter for 2–3 minutes on each side, or until the pineapple is charred and deep golden coloured. Repeat the process with the remaining pineapple.

4. Place the cooked pineapple pieces on a platter and pour over the spiced ginger and black pepper syrup. Serve immediately, with frozen yoghurt if you wish.

 Time Saving Hack
You can use tinned pineapple rings in this recipe, provided you drain and pat dry with kitchen paper before using.

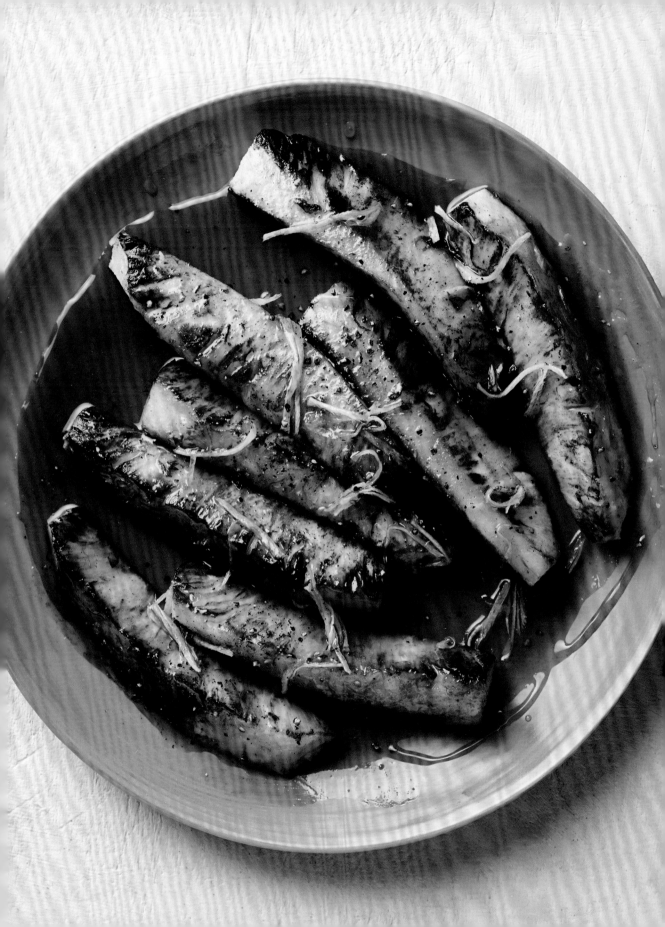

Melon Ribbons with Sumac

Diversity points: 5 / Fibre: 4.3g

½ small cantaloupe melon

½ small honeydew melon

Juice of 1 clementine/tangerine

3 tbsp pomegranate seeds

1 generous tbsp sumac

Handful of mint leaves

Pinch of sea salt

+ Bonus Diversity Points

Serve the melon salad studded with blueberries and toasted almonds.

Magical melon, ripe and sweet at its peak, is a real treat when dusted with sour, fruity sumac and fresh mint. I use honeydew and cantaloupe melon here, but you can other fruits of your choice, like nectarines and plums or oranges and grapefruit.

1. Remove the seeds from both types of melon and cut them into thick wedges, then use a potato peeler to cut the melon into thin strips. If the melon is too ripe and can't be cut into thin strips, don't worry, just chop it into 2cm (¾in) dice. Discard the melon skin.

2. Scatter the melon ribbons over a large platter and squeeze over the juice from the clementine. Sprinkle over the pomegranate seeds and sumac, then tear the mint leaves and strew them over the melon. Sprinkle a little salt over the melon before serving.

 ### Time Saving Hack
You can have the melon ready in the fridge beforehand. Just top with the clementine juice, sumac, mint and salt before serving. Buy pre-cut fruit if you are very time-stretched.

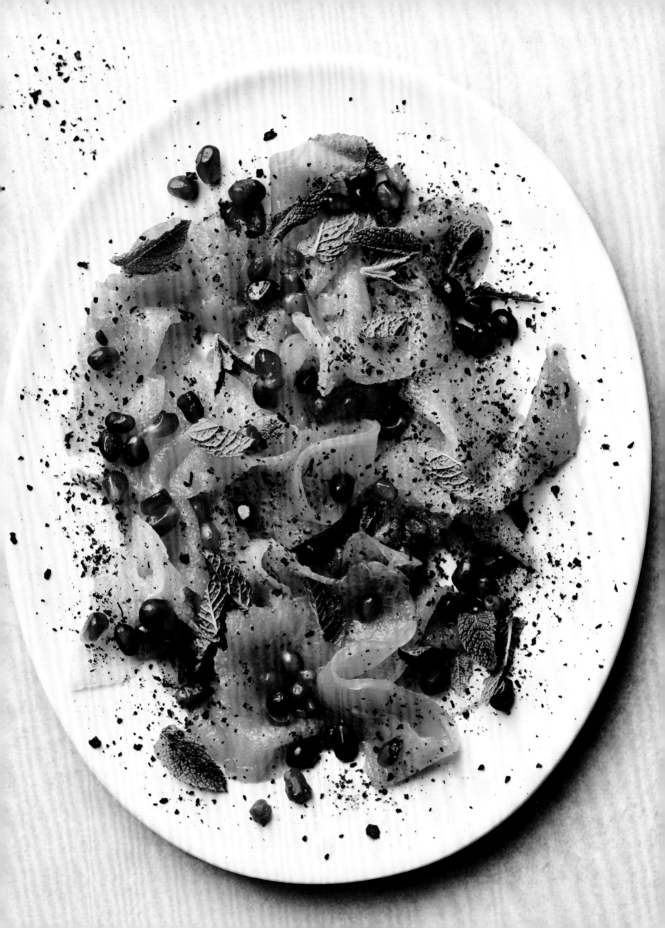

Index

Note: page numbers in **bold** refer to illustrations.

Thanks

Pinch me please! Writing the acknowledgements for my fourth book. Who could have thought? I strongly believe that people never do exist in isolation, we are all defined by community, and no woman is an island. All my success to date is testament to the hard work of all those who have chosen to surround me with their unwavering love and support.

My husband Usman Ahmed has been the subject of all my food experiments and my late night companion, supporting 'The 20-Minute Gut Fix' since its very inception. I am eternally grateful for his support as a father to our children as I pursue my writing. I love that you love my success and I love everything you succeed with too.

Nicky Ross, editor extraordinaire and the woman who makes thing happen for me. You are truly incredible, and I would be nowhere without your clear vision for my books and writing. You are yin to my writing yang and the apple of my writing eye. I am eternally grateful to Elly James and Heather Holden Brown of HHB agency for making our relationship ever stronger and fostering my writing so beautifully... as friends more than agents.

A huge thank you also to my brother, Taha Mahmood who was one of my chief taste testers – best brother in the world, no honestly, mine is elite. Once again, a special mention to Sheriar Arjani, who took the time to go through and edit my entire manuscript, you are the best of writing companions and I so wish that one day this becomes a full time job for you, you are so good at it! And dare I say, funnier than me.

Next, a huge thanks to the whole team at Hodder books, in particular Charlotte Macdonald and Olivia Nightingall; seamless passage of the torch and such beautiful organisation, made my life so darn easy. Alainna Hadjigeorgiou, I am eternally grateful for all your tireless graft, meticulous planning making my work known to the wider world. Sumptuous, effortless food photography from Steven Joyce, supported by Lizzie Harris' expert styling and Max Robinson's props – you are a man of good taste! Steve, I really cherish all the memories we made together in Kemble House studios, as those Polaroid shots slowly came together against the side wall. I miss our conversations over shoot lunches already. Nikki at Nic & Lou design studio, well I mean the book speaks for itself. I'm always blown away by how you understand my creative vision and make it come to fruition effortlessly. The book is edible!! Which is the best compliment that a cookbook could have.

Finally, thank you for picking this book up and reading it, cooking from it and making it a part of your life. Books are living entities, that you find joy and comfort in mine is the biggest compliment this humble author could ever have.

First published in Great Britain in 2025 by Yellow Kite
An imprint of Hodder & Stoughton
An Hachette UK company
1

Hardback ISBN: 9781399735971
eBook ISBN: 9781399735988

Editorial Director: Nicky Ross
Project Editor: Charlotte Macdonald
Design and illustration : Studio Nic&Iou
Photography: Steven Joyce
Food Stylist: Lizzie Harris
Props Stylist: Max Robinson
Senior Production Controller: Claudette Morris

Colour origination by Alta
Printed and bound in China by C&C Offset Printing Co., Ltd.
Hodder & Stoughton policy is to use papers that are natural, renewable and recyclable products
and made from wood grown in sustainable forests. The logging and manufacturing processes
are expected to conform to the environmental regulations of the country of origin.W

Yellow Kite
Hodder & Stoughton Ltd
Carmelite House
50 Victoria Embankment
London
EC4Y 0DZ

www.yellowkitebooks.co.uk
www.hodder.co.uk

Notes
The information and references contained herein are for informational purposes only. They are designed to support, not replace, any ongoing medical advice given by a healthcare professional and should not be construed as the giving of medical advice nor relied upon as a basis for any decision or action. Readers should consult their doctor before altering their diet, particularly if they are on a set diet prescribed by their doctor or dietician. The fibre count for each recipe is an estimate only and may vary depending on the brand of ingredients used, and due to the natural biological variations in the composition of foods such as meat, fish, fruit and vegetables. It does not include the nutritional content of garnishes or any optional accompaniments recommended for taste/serving in the ingredients list.